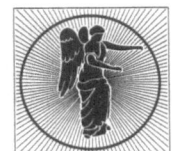

Bi & Gi Publishers

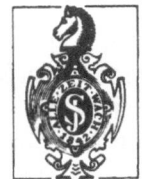

Current Topics in Rehabilitation
Series Editor : R. Corsico M.D.

Titles in the series:

Respiratory Muscles in Chronic Obstructive Pulmonary Disease
Edited by: A. Grassino, C. Fracchia, C. Rampulla, L. Zocchi

Pathophysiology and Treatment of Pulmonary Circulation
Edited by: A. Morpurgo, R. Tramarin, C. Rampulla, C. Fracchia, F. Cobelli

Chronic Pulmonary Hyperinflation
Edited by: A. Grassino, C. Rampulla, N. Ambrosino, C. Fracchia

Biochemistry of Pulmonary Emphysema
Edited by: C. Grassi, J. Travis, L. Casali, M. Luisetti

Nutrition and Ventilatory Function
Edited by: R.D. Ferranti, C. Rampulla, C. Fracchia, N. Ambrosino

Forthcoming titles in the series:

Pulmonary Rehabilitation
Edited by: A. Grassino, C. Fracchia, C. Rampulla

Acknowledgments: this volume contains a selection of papers presented at the International Symposium "Pulmonary Circulation V", Prague, July 5-7 1989, in the sessions on: "Right ventricular hypertrophy" and "Clinical estimation of right ventricular function".
The Organizing Commitee gratefully acknowledges the Clinica del Lavoro Foundation, Pavia (Italy), for their support and co-operation.

Right Ventricular Hypertrophy and Function in Chronic Lung Disease

Edited by: V. Ježek, M. Morpurgo, R. Tramarin

Foreword by: R. Corsico
With 58 figures and 49 tables

Springer-Verlag London Ltd.

V. Ježek   Institute of Physiological Regulations, Czechoslovak Academy of Sciences, Prague, Czechoslovakia
M. Morpurgo   Department of Cardiology, S. Carlo Borromeo Hospital, Milan, Italy
R. Tramarin   Division of Cardiology, Clinica del Lavoro Foundation, Institute of Care and Research, Medical Center of Rehabilitation, Montescano, Pavia, Italy

Series Editor:
R. Corsico   Clinica del Lavoro Foundation, Institute of Care and Research, Medical Center of Rehabilitation, Montescano, Pavia, Italy

ISBN 978-1-4471-3855-6
British Library Cataloguing in Publication Data
Right Ventricular Hypertrophy and Function in Chronic Lung Disease. - (Current Topics in Rehabilitation Series) I. Jezek, Vlastimil II. Series 616.2
ISBN 978-1-4471-3855-6   ISBN 978-1-4471-3853-2 (eBook)
DOI 10.1007/978-1-4471-3853-2

Library of Congress Cataloging-in- Publication Data
Right Ventricular Hypertrophy and Function in Chronic Lung Disease / edited by V. Jezek, M. Morpurgo, R. Tramarin; foreword by R. Corsico.
p. cm. — (Current topics in rehabilitation) Includes index.
ISBN 978-1-4471-3855-6
1. Heart—Right ventricle—Hypertrophy. 2. Lungs—Diseases. Obstructive—Complications. 3. Lung Diseases. Obstructive—physiopathology. I. Jezek, V. (Vlastimil), 1934-II. Morpurgo, M. (Mario), 1925-. III, Tramarin, R. (Roberto), 1951-IV Series.
(DNLM: 1. Heart Enlargement—physiopatology. 2. Lung Diseases, Obstructive—aetiology. WG 200 R571) RC685.H9R54 1992. 616, 1'2—dc20
DNLM/DLC for Library of Congress 92-2330 CIP

Typeset by Bi & Gi, Verona, Italy

Preface

This monograph comprises 17 papers written by prominent authors in the field, each of whom presents his most recent experiences. The papers were not specially selected so that this work is far from being a comprehensive textbook covering all aspects of right ventricular hypertrophy and failure in chronic lung disease.

Perhaps some of the papers dealing with more strictly physiological problems and experimental models will be somewhat difficult to relate directly to former modes of thinking of both cardiologists and pneumologists. Nevertheless, we hope and expect that this book will provide the reader with, an in-depth appreciation of the situation of present research in different laboratories and countries.

Occasionally contradictions between different papers may be noticed. We have not tried to remove these, since each contradiction reflects current areas of dispute or uncertainty in this developing field.

We wish finally to acknowledge the continuing support of the Clinica del Lavoro Foundation for projects aimed at promoting education in all fields related to medical rehabilitation.

Vlastimil Ježek
Mario Morpurgo
Roberto Tramarin

Foreword

This volume is the sixth issue in the Series "Current Topics in Rehabilitation", which was first conceived in 1987 with the aim of offering updated indications as to functional comprehensive evaluation strategies and rehabilitation programmes. One particular feature of the book is that we decided it would be worthwhile adopting an interdisciplinary approach to cardiopulmonary aspects. We trust that the notion that "pulmonary circulation is a kind of no-man's land between pulmonology and cardiology for everyone except physiologists" (H. Denolin, 1988) is now virtually a thing of the past.

Thus, despite the fact that most of the topics addressed in this book deal with strictly physiopathological problems, we believe that they may make a substantial speculative contribution to the work of both for pneumologists and cardiologists who, in the clinical context, find themselves having to cope with situations related to cor pulmonale and right ventricular hypertrophy.

May 1992

RENATO CORSICO

Contents

X

Contributors

ALLI C.
Vergani Medical Division, Niguarda Cà Granda Hospital, Milan, Italy

ALPAGO R.
Cardiology Department, Niguarda Cà Granda Hospital, Milan, Italy

APPRILL M.
Pulmonary Function Laboratory, Pavillon Laennec, University Hospital, Strasbourg, France

BASS A.
Institute of Physiology, Czechoslovak Academy of Sciences, Kardiocentrum, Faculty Hospital Motol and Department of Cardiology, Postgraduate Medical School, Prague, Czechoslovakia

BERTOLI L.
Vergani Medical Division, Niguarda Cà Granda Hospital, Milan, Italy

BURGHUBER O.C.
Second Medical Department, University of Vienna, Austria

CIHAK R.
Department of Cardiology, Postgraduate Medical and Pharmaceutical Institute, Czechoslovak Academy of Sciences, Prague, Czechoslovakia

DEES A.
Department of Internal Medicine, Ikaziaziekenhuis and Zuiderziekenhuis, Rotterdam, Netherlands

DE LEEUW P.W.
Department of Internal Medicine, Zuiderziekenhuis, Rotterdam, Netherlands

DENOLIN H.
Department of Cardiology, Saint-Pierre University Hospital, Brussels, Belgium

DOLENSKY J.
Department of Tuberculosis and Respiratory Diseases, Thomayer's Teaching Hospital, Prague, Czechoslovakia

EHRHART M.
Pulmonary Function Laboratory, Pavillon Laennec, University Hospital, Strasbourg, France

FAULKNER C.S.
Department of Physiology, Pathology, Pharmacology and Toxicology, Dartmouth Medical School, Hanover, NH, USA

HAMMER J.
Department of Medicine, Institute for Clinical and Experimental Medicine, Prague, Czechoslovakia

HAWRYLKIEWICZ I.
Department of Respiratory Medicine, Institute of Tuberculosis and Lung Disease, University Hospital, Warsaw, Poland
HENRIQUEZ A.
CHU Brabois, Vandoeuvre, Nancy, France
HEYSTEEG M.
Department of Pulmonary Medicine, Zuiderziekenhuis, Rotterdam, Netherlands
HILL N.S.
Pulmonary Division, Rhode Island Hospital, Providence, RI, USA
JEŽEK V.
Institute of Physiological Regulations, Czechoslovak Academy of Sciences, Prague, Czechoslovakia
JEŽKOVA J.
Institute of Physiological Regulations, Czechoslovak Academy of Sciences, Prague, Czechoslovakia
KOLAR F.
Institute of Physiology, Czechoslovak Academy of Sciences, Kardiocentrum, Faculty Hospital Motol and Department of Cardiology, Postgraduate Medical School, Prague, Czechoslovakia
KROFTA K.
Department of Tuberculosis and Respiratory Diseases, Thomayer's Teaching Hospital, Prague, Czechoslovakia
MACNEE W.
Department of Respiratory Medicine, City Hospital, Edinburgh, UK
MAMMOSSER M.O.
Pulmonary Function Laboratory, Pavillon Laennec, University Hospital, Strasbourg, France
MANTERO A.
Cardiology Department, Niguarda Cà Granda Hospital, Milan, Italy
MICHALJANIC A.
Institute of Physiological Regulations, Czechoslovak Academy of Sciences, Prague, Czechoslovakia
MILEROVA M.
Institute of Physiology, Czechoslovak Academy of Sciences, Kardiocentrum, Faculty Hospital Motol and Department of Cardiology, Postgraduate Medical School, Prague, Czechoslovakia
MIRHOM R.
Pulmonary Function Laboratory, Pavillon Laennec, University Hospital, Strasbourg, France
MISKIEWICZ Z.
Department of Hypertension and Angiology, Academy of Medicine, Warsaw, Poland
MOLINO A.
Vergani Medical Division, Niguarda Cà Granda Hospital, Milan, Italy

MORPURGO M.
Department of Cardiology, S. Carlo Borromeo Hospital, Milan, Italy

NIEDERLE P.
Institute of Physiological Regulations, Czechoslovak Academy of Sciences, Prague, Czechoslovakia

OSTADAL B.
Institute of Physiology, Czechoslovak Academy of Sciences, Kardiocentrum, Faculty Hospital Motol and Department of Cardiology, Postgraduate Medical School, Prague, Czechoslovakia

OU L.C.
Department of Physiology, Pathology, Pharmacology and Toxicology, Dartmouth Medical School, Hanover, NH, USA

PASIERSKI T.
Department of Hypertension and Angiology, Academy of Medicine, Warsaw, Poland

PELOUCH V.
Institute of Physiology, Czechoslovak Academy of Sciences, Kardiocentrum, Faculty Hospital Motol and Department of Cardiology, Postgraduate Medical School, Prague, Czechoslovakia

PEZZANO A.
Cardiology Department, Niguarda Cà Granda Hospital, Milan, Italy

PICKETT B.P.
Department of Physiology, Pathology, Pharmacology and Toxicology, Dartmouth Medical School, Hanover, NH, USA

POLU J.M.
CHU Brabois, Vandoeuvre, Nancy, France

PROCHAZKA J.
Institute of Physiology, Czechoslovak Academy of Sciences, Kardiocentrum, Faculty Hospital Motol and Department of Cardiology, Postgraduate Medical School, Prague, Czechoslovakia

REDONDO J.
CHU Brabois, Vandoeuvre, Nancy, France

SARDELLA G.L.
Department of Physiology, Pathology, Pharmacology and Toxicology, Dartmouth Medical School, Hanover, NH, USA

SCHRIJEN F.
INSERM, Unit 14, Vandoeuvre, Nancy, France

SKWARSKI K.
Department of Respiratory Medicine, City Hospital, Edinburgh, UK

SKWARSKI K.
Department of Respiratory Medicine, Institute of Tuberculosis and Lung Disease, University Hospital, Warsaw, Poland

TAMPONI M.
Physical Therapy Department, Niguarda Cà Granda Hospital, Milan, Italy

TENNEY S.M.
Department of Physiology, Pathology, Pharmacology and Toxicology, Dartmouth Medical School, Hanover, NH, USA

THRON C.D.
Department of Physiology, Pathology, Pharmacology and Toxicology, Dartmouth Medical School, Hanover, NH, USA

TORBICKI A.
Department of Hypertension and Angiology, Academy of Medicine Warsaw, Poland

TRAMARIN R.
Division of Cardiology, Clinica del Lavoro Foundation, Institute of Care and Research, Medical Center of Rehabilitation, Montescano (Pavia) Italy

VAN ES P.N.
Department of Internal Medicine, Zuiderziekenhuis, Rotterdam, Netherlands

WEITZENBLUM E.
Pulmonary Function Laboratory, University Hospital, Pavillon Laennec, Strasbourg, France

WIDIMSKY J.
Institute of Physiology, Czechoslovak Academy of Sciences, Kardiocentrum, Faculty Hospital Motol and Department of Cardiology, Postgraduate Medical School, Prague, Czechoslovakia

ZIELINSKI J.
Department of Respiratory Medicine, Institute of Tuberculosis and Lung Disease, University Hospital, Warsaw, Poland

1. Right Heart Failure in Chronic Lung Disease. Where Are We Now?

V. JEŽEK,[1] M. MORPURGO[2]

1. *Institute of Physiological Regulations, Czechoslovak Academy of Sciences, Prague, Czechoslovakia*
2. *Department of Cardiology, S. Carlo Borromeo Hospital, Milan, Italy*

There is no uniformity in the definition of cardiac failure and all authors agree that a generally valuable definition is extremely difficult. An attempt of five outstanding cardiologists was published in 1983[1] with following discussion and criticism of other experts:[2-4]

"Heart failure is the state of any heart disease in which, despite adequate ventricular filling, the heart's output is decreased or in which the heart is unable to pump blood at a rate adequate for satisfying the requirements of the tissues with function parameters remaining within normal limits."

Some cardiologists use a more or less similar definition;[5,6,9] others include also the state of peripheral circulation and tissue metabolism in the definition.[7,8,10]

When the clinicians see these definitions of cardiac failure they feel instinctively that something is missing here: a link describing intermediate cases between the normality and frank failure. It concerns e.g. the cases with normal haemodynamics at rest but with abnormal reaction under stress - during exercise or in abnormal pressure or volume load. Another example could be the presence of a frank haemodynamic abnormality at rest but without clinical signs of failure. Similar situation could be called "cardiac dysfunction" or "abnormal cardiac function".[6]

The descriptions of a clinical and haemodynamic picture of Right Heart Failure (RHF) in chronic lung disease[11-16] emphasize that RHF differs substantially from the usual features of cardiac failure encountered e.g. in ischaemic or valvular heart disease. First, the cardiac output is usually normal. Second, the reaction of peripheral circulation is different; there is no vasoconstriction.

These findings have led various investigators to the reflection whether oedema in RHF is purely of "cardiac" origin. Two mechanisms were particularly accused of participation: the direct effect of hypoxia on the permeability of vascular wall[17,19] and altered renal function.

Renal function in RHF was studied as early as in 1951.[20,21] Following studies can be briefly summarized as follows:

a. There is a consistent decrease of renal blood flow in the phase of oedema[20-25] which is followed by an increase during the diuretic phase.
b. No consistent conclusion could be drawn for the behaviour of electrolytes, particularly Na^+ and K^+. Most authors found that their changes differ from those observed in cardiac failure secondary to ischaemic or valvular disease.[26-29] The differences are usually attributed to the presence of hypoxaemia and to the need for the buffering of hypercarbic acidosis but the results regarding the relation of blood gases to electrolyte retention and excretion are often controversial.[20-23]
c. The presence of oedema is not associated with significant increase of body weight and total body water.[30] There is a loss of body weight during the diuretic phase and slow subsequent regain of weight during the convalescence. These changes are probably at least partly associated with the changes of tissue proteins and not only to those of the water itself[30] and are also related to the changes of K^+ metabolism.[31]

We have only little data about humoral changes (renin-aldosterone complex, etc.) in RHF secondary to lung disease.

In conclusion, the definition and description of RHF secondary to lung diseases is not easy. From the haemodynamic point of view it corresponds rather to the classification of "abnormal cardiac function" than failure and we find numerous differences (haemodynamic and metabolic) in regard to the cardiac failure of "classical" type (ischaemic or valvular origin).

There is also a further definition which deserves critical discussion - the term "cor pulmonale".

This term, introduced probably by Paul D. White in 1931 was defined by the WHO Expert Committee[32] as "hypertrophy of the right ventricle resulting from diseases affecting the function and/or structure of the lungs, except when these pulmonary alterations are the result of diseases that primarily affect the left side of the heart, as in congenital heart disease".

Already at first sight this definition has very limited clinical value since the Right Ventricular (RV) hypertrophy could be exactly recognized only at autopsy; all noninvasive methods are not sufficiently sensitive.[33]

Similar definition was used by Behnke et al.[34]; only the expression "hypertrophy" was replaced by "alteration in structure or function of the right ventricle". We see that this definition covers "all that is not entirely normal" from mild RV hypertrophy with normal cardiac function to frank RHF. We feel that this spectrum is too large to be useful for the clinician.

Furthermore, other authors often use the term "cor pulmonale" as a synonym for RHF.[13,15,16]

All these definitions exist in the present literature and could introduce serious bias into the clinical classification of patients.

We propose therefore to abandon completely the term "cor pulmonale" and to speak only about RV hypertrophy, enlargement, functional abnormality or failure provided we have objective evidence for such a statement.

Many authors have described significant differences regarding global haemodynamic values between the patients with and without clinical signs of RHF[35-40]: the latter group exhibits lower resting and exertional right atrial and pulmonary arterial pressure and lower pulmonary vascular resistance. The cardiac output is almost the same in both subgroups: it is normal on the average and it rises during low-level exercise[37-42] proportionally to the results obtained in healthy subjects of comparable age.[43-44]

All authors describe a large scatter of individual haemodynamic values and their overlap between the subgroups. Further, the pulmonary arterial pressure and vascular resistance are rather labile according to the state of respiration.[45-47] Moreover, normal cardiac output has been found in patients with COLD but not e.g. in so-called primary pulmonary hypertension[48-50] and probably not in terminal stages of some other lung diseases (Jezek et al. in this volume).

It is therefore practically impossible to decide about the state of right ventricular function from global haemodynamic values.

The classification of RV function should be done in more exact terms and we are obliged to distinguish between the pump function and contractility. We must also realize that the examination of the RV could be technically more difficult than the same approach used for the left ventricle.[51-54] These questions are analysed in more detail elsewhere (Morpurgo and Jezek in this volume).

There is also one important haemodynamic circumstance which is rarely mentioned: tricuspid regurgitation.

Its importance has been outlined quite recently.[55-57] The incidence of tricuspid regurgitation in chronic lung disease is relatively high.[57,58] It decreases substantially resulting cardiac output[55-59] and it compromises also the reliability of RV ejection fraction as a measure of the pump function.[60]

A practical application of different methods of investigation shows that radionuclide ventriculography is the most widely used and satisfactorily compared with the reference methods.

The other approaches like echocardiography[61-67] (Niederle et al. in this volume) and thermodilution[68] for the measurement of RV ejection fraction seem to be very promising but up till now not so widely used.

The recognition of early stages of RV dysfunction remains the field for further research. The incapacity of the right ventricle to increase its ejection fraction in exercise seems to be informative (see also Schrijen et al. in this volume).

The first communications dealing with the prognosis of chronic lung disease (CLD) in general and clinical signs of RHF in particular are from the 1960s. It has been described that the mean time from the first appearance of the signs of RHF till death varies from 1.3 to 3.8 years.[69-73]

Many authors tried to relate the mortality in CLD rather to more exactly classified results of functional tests than to the signs of RHF. In particular, spirography and blood gases have been proved to be significantly related to patients' survival.[71-79] Most papers emphasized that the presence and degree of pulmonary hypertension is most closely related to the prognosis.[73,80-84] It concerns not only COLD but also other lung diseases: silicosis[85,86], interstitial lung fibrosis[87,88], tuberculosis[86] and thromboembolic disease.[89] It corresponds also to the results of our WHO cooperative study.[90] The only exception is probably so-called "primary" PH in which no relation between the degree of PH and survival has been found.[91-94]

It has been felt that the correlations with PH, i.e. with RV pressure overload, represent also the relation between RV failure and mortality. To our surprise, the first studies dealing with this problem have found only a weak correlation between RV ejection fraction and mortality.[95,96]

Some authors have thought decreased tissue oxygen delivery to be more closely related to the vital prognosis in CLD than PH and RHF.[98-99] However, tissue oxygen delivery seems to be preserved in most cases of COLD (Jezek et al. in this volume); hypoxaemia is compensated by normal cardiac output even in most advanced stages of the disease.

Therefore, the influence of individual functional parameters in CLD on vital prognosis remains quite obscure. Some authors[100] always believed that no individual factor from the complexity present in underlying disease could satisfactorily express the prognosis.

Also the direct cause of death in CLD is not entirely clear. Certainly it is not the cardiac failure in the sense which we encounter it in left heart disease; it is difficult to imagine a "real" cardiac failure with normal cardiac output.

Some authors outlined a high incidence of pulmonary embolism and thromboembolic disease in patients with CLD.[97,101,103] However, most authors believe that a majority of emboli found at autopsy are terminal.

The incidence of malignant arrhythmias is often discussed[104] (Dolensky et al. in this volume) but the group of examined patients is not sufficiently large for a definite conclusion.

There is no doubt that most patients with advanced COLD have a serious metabolic disorder; the mechanism of death should probably be sought there. More detailed data are however lacking.

One possible source of limitation of our knowledge about the mechanisms of death in CLD is one defect which appears in most studies. They could be divided in two subgroups: the first one includes the patients with very good clinical and functional characteristics but the number of autopsies is low. The second subgroup consists of well documented autopsies accompanied by limited clinical data.

RHF in CLD seems to be a complex event which must not be simplified only to RV pressure overload and/or the blood gas disturbance. Its specific features are particularly the normal myocardial contractility and the ability to maintain normal cardiac output almost till death. The reason for it, as well as for other differences from usual picture of heart failure in left heart disease, is not satisfactorily elucidated.

Our knowledge of the terminal mechanisms by which RHF contributes to death in patients with CLD is very limited.

References

1. Denolin H., Kuhn H., Krayenbuehl HP., Loogen F., Reale A.: The definition of heart failure. Eur. Heart J. 1983; 4:445-448
2. Julian DG.: Comment to preceding article. Eur. Heart J. 1983;4:446
3. Braunwald E.: Comment to preceding article. Eur. Heart J. 1983;4:446-7
4. Gibson DG.: Comment to preceding article. Eur. Heart J. 1983;4:447-8
5. Braunwald E., Mock MM., Watson JT.: Congestive heart failure: A propitious time for intensified research. Am. J. Cardiol. 1983;51:603-10
6. Braunwald E.: Pathophysiology of heart failure. In: E. Braunwald, (Ed.) *Heart diseases*, Philadelphia, Saunders 1980; p. 453-471.
7. Poole-Wilson PA.: Heart failure. Med. Int. 1985;2:866-871
8. Poole-Wilson PA.: The origin of symptoms in patients with chronic heart failure. Eur. Heart J. 1988;9 (Suppl H): 49-53
9. Taylor SH.: Cardiovascular consequences of heart failure. Eur. Heart J. 1988; 9 (Suppl H): 41-47
10. Jezek V.: Vasodilator treatment in cardiac and pulmonary patients. In: M. Morpurgo, R. Tramarin, C. Rampulla, C. Fracchia and F. Cobelli (Eds.), *Pathophysiology and treatment of pulmonary circulation*, Bi & Gi, Springer, 1988; p. 139-145.
11. Harris P., Heath D.: *The human pulmonary circulation*, Edinburgh, Livingstone, 1977; p. 522-546.
12. Howard P.: Aetiological factors in hypoxic cor pulmonale. Prog. Resp. Res. 1985; 20:49-54
13. Rubin J.L.: Pulmonary hypertension secondary to lung disease. In: EK Weir and JT Reeves (Eds.),*Pulmonary hypertension*, New York, Futura, 1984; p. 291-320.
14. McFadden E.R., Braunwald E.: Cor pulmonale and pulmonary thromboembolism. In: E. Braunwald, *Heart diseases*, (Ed.) Philadelphia, Saunders, 1980; p. 453-471.
15. Hooper R.G.: Chronic right heart failure: Pulmonary considerations. In: R.L. Fisk (Ed.), *The right heart*, Philadelphia, Davis 1987; p. 181-190.
16. Wiedemann HP., Matthay RA.: The management of acute and chronic cor pulmonale. In: SM. Scharf and SS Cassidy (Ed.),*Heart-lung interactions in health and disease*, New York, Dekker, 1989; p. 915-982.
17. Parker R.E., Granger D.N., Taylor A.E.: Estimates of isogravimetric capillary pressures during

6

alveolar hypoxia. Am. J. Physiol. 1981;241:H732-H739

18. Schoene R.B., Hackett P.H., Henderson W.R. et al: High altitude pulmonary edema. Characteristics of lung lavage fluid. J. Am. Med. Ass. 1986; 256:63-69
19. Kinasewitz G.T, Groome J.L, Marchall R.P., Leslie W.K., Diana J.N.: Effect of hypoxia on permeability of pulmonary endothelium of canine visceral pleura. J. Appl. Physiol. 1986; 61:554-560
20. Fishman A.P., Maxwell M.H., Crowder C.H., Morales P.: Kidney function in cor pulmonale. Circulation 1951;3:703-721
21. Davies C.E.: Renal circulation in cor pulmonale. Lancet 1951; 2, 1052-1057
22. Stuart-Harris C.H., MacKinnon J., Hamond J.D.S., Smith D.W.: The renal circulation in chronic pulmonary disease and pulmonary heart failure. Quart .J. Med. 1956; 25:389-405
23. Aber G.M., Bishop J.M.: Serial changes in renal function, arterial gas tensions and the acid-base state in patients with chronic bronchitis and oedema. Clin. Sci. 1965;28:511-525
24. Platts M.M., Hammond J.D.S., Stuart-Harris C.H.: A study of cor pulmonale in patients with chronic bronchitis. Quart. J. Med. 1960; 29:559-574
25. Richens J.M., Howard P.: Oedema in cor pulmonale. Clin. Sci. 1982; 62:255-259
26. Aikawa J.K., Fitz R.H.: Alterations in exchangeable sodium content, sodium space and body weight during the treatment of congestive failure. Circulation 1955; 12:897-902
27. Birkenfeld L.W., Leibman J., O'Meara M.P., Edelman I.S.: Total exchangeable sodium, total exchangeable potassium and total body water in oedematous patients with cirrhosis of the liver and congestive heart failure. J. Clin. Invest. 1958; 37:687-698
28. Mader K.H., Morita Y., Iseri L.T.: Sodium, potassium and magnesium balance during recovery from congestive heart failure due to cor pulmonale and other heart disease. Circulation 1955; 12:1057-1064
29. Cox J.R., Horrocks P., Speight C.J., Pearson R.E., Hobson N.: Potassium and sodium distribution in cardiac failure. Clin. Sci. 1971;41:55-61
30. Campbell R.H.A., Brand H.L., Cox J.R., Howard P.: Body weight and body water in chronic cor pulmonale. Clin. Sci. Mol. Med. 1975; 49:323-335
31. Morgan D.B., Burkinshaw L., Davidson C.: Potassium depletion in heart failure and its relation to long term treatment with diuretics: a review of the literature. Postgrad. Med. J. 1978;54:72-79
32. World Health Organization. Chronic cor pulmonale: Report of an expert committee. Circulation 1963;27:594-615
33. Jezek V., Denolin H., Weitzenblum E., Morpurgo M.: Noninvasive diagnosis of pulmonary hypertension in chronic lung disease revisited. Eur. Respir. J. (in press)
34. Behnke R.H, Blount S.G., Bristow J.D., Carrieri V., Pierce J.A., Sasahara A., Soffer A.:Primary prevention of pulmonary heart disease. Circulation 1970;41:A17-A23
35. Williams J.F., Behnke R.H.: The effect of pulmonary emphysema upon cardiopulmonary hemodynamics at rest and during exercise. Ann. Intern. Med. 1964;60:824-842
36. Herles F., Jezek V., Daum S.: Site of pulmonary resistance in cor pulmonale in chronic bronchitis. Br. Heart J. 1968;30:654-660
37. Horsfield K., Segel N., Bishop J.M.: The pulmonary circulation in chronic bronchitis at rest and during exercise breathing air and 80% oxygen. Clin. Sci. 1968;43:473-483
38. Lockhart A., Tzareva M., Nader F., Leblanc P., Schrijen F., Sadoul P.: Elevated pulmonary artery wedge pressure at rest and during exercise in chronic bronchitis: Fact or fancy. Clin. Sci. 1969; 37:503-517
39. Jezek V., Schrijen F.: Haemodynamic effect of deslanoside at rest and during exercise in patients with chronic bronchitis. Br. Heart J. 1973; 35:2-8
40. Jezek V., Schrijen F., Sadoul P.: Right ventricular function and pulmonary hemodynamics during

exercise in patients with chronic obstructive pulmonary disease. Cardiology 1973;58:20-31

41. Light R.W., Mintz H.M., Linden G.S., Brown S.E.: Hemodynamics of patients with severe chronic obstructive pulmonary disease during progressive upright exercise. Am Rev. Resp. Dis. 1984;130:391-395

42. Weitzenblum E., El Charbic T., Vanderenne A., Blegar A., Hirth C., Oudet P.: Pulmonary haemodynamic changes during muscular exercise in non-decompensated chronic bronchitis. Bull. Physiopath. Resp. 1972;8:49-71

43. Granath A., Jansson B., Strandell T.: Circulation in healthy old men studied by right heart catheterization at rest and during exercise in supine and sitting position. Acta Med. Scand. 1964;176:425-426

44. Holmgren A., Jansson B., Sjöstrand T.: Circulatory data in normal subjects at rest and during exercise in recumbent position with special reference to the stroke volume at different work intensities. Acta Physiol. Scand. 1960;49:343-363

45. Jezek V., Ouredník A.: Development of pulmonary hypertension in chronic cor pulmonale and emphysema; Its relationship to the development of chronic respiratory insufficiency. Bull. Physiopath. Resp. 1968;4:297-305

46. Jezek V., Michaljanic A., Fucík J., Ramaisl R.: Long-term development of pulmonary arterial pressure in diffuse interstitial lung fibrosis. Prog. Respir. Res. 1985;20:170-175

47. Weitzenblum E., Jezek V.: Evolution of pulmonary hypertension in chronic respiratory diseases. Bull. Eur. Physiopath. Resp. 1984;20: 73-81

48. Rich S., Levy P.S.: Characteristics of surviving and nonsurviving patients with primary pulmonary hypertension. Am. J. Med. 1984;76:573-578

49. Rozkovec A., Montanez P., Oakley C.M.: Factors that influence the outcome of primary pulmonary hypertension. Br. Heart J. 1986; 55:449-458

50. Fuster V., Steel P.M., Edwards W.D et al.: Primary pulmonary hypertension: Favorable effect of isoproterenol. New Engl. J. Med. 1976;295:1414-1415

51. Maughan W.L., Oikawa R.Y.: Right ventricular function. In: S.M. Scharf and S.S Cassidy (Ed.), *Heart-lung interactions in health and disease*, New York, Dekker, 1989; p. 179-220.

52. Morris J.J., Wechsler A.S.: Right ventricular function: the assessment of contractile performance. In: R.L. Fick (Ed.),*The right heart*, Philadelphia, Davis, 1987; p. 3-18.

53. Morrison D.A., Harnett S.D., Adcock K.: Radionuclide and angiographic assessment of the right heart. In: R.L. Fick (Ed.), *The right heart*, Philadelphia, Davis, 1987; p. 19-32.

54. Oboler A.A., Keefe J.F., Gaasch W.H., Banas J.S., Levine H.J.: Influence of left ventricular isovolumic pressure upon right ventricular pressure transients. Cardiology 1973;58:30-44

55. Wooley L.F.: Rediscovery of the tricuspid valve. Curr. Probl. Cardiovasc. Dis. 1981;6:7-41

56. Ubago J.L., Figuero A., Ochoteco A., Colman T., Duran R.M., Duran C.G.: Analysis of the amount of tricuspid valve annular dilatation required to produce functional tricuspid regurgitation. Am. J. Cardiol. 1983;52:155-158

57. Waller B.F.: Etiology of pure tricuspid regurgitation. In: R.L. Fisk (Ed.), *The right heart*, Philadelphia, Davis, 1987; p. 53-95.

58. Hansing C.E., Rowe G.C.: Tricuspid insufficiency: a study of hemodynamics and pathogenesis. Circulation 1972;45:793-801

59. Schwartz F., Manthey J., Schuler G et al: The effect of tricuspid insufficiency on right ventricular performance in patients with valvular heart disease. Z. Kardiol. 1981;70:466-503

60. Morrison D.A., Ovitt T., Hammermeister K.E.: Functional tricuspid regurgitation and right ventricular dysfunction in pulmonary hypertension. Am. J. Cardiol. 1988; 62:108-112

61. Kaul S., Tei C., Hopkins J.M., Shah P.M.: Assessment of right ventricular function using two-dimensional echocardiography. Am. Heart J. 1984;107:526-531

8

62. Gibson T.C., Miller S.W., Aretz T., Hardin N.J., Weyman AE.: Method for estimating right ventricular volume by planes applicable to cross-sectional echocardiography: correlation with angiographic formulas. Am. J. Cardiol. 1985;55:1584-1588

63. Panidis I.P., Ren J.F., Kotler M.N., Mintz G., Iskandrian A., Ross J., Kane S.: Two-dimensional echocardiographic estimation of right ventricular ejection fraction in patients with coronary artery disease. J. Am. Coll. Cardiol. 1983;2:911-918

64. Levine R.A., Gibson T.C., Aretz T., Gillam L.D., Guyer D.E., King M.E., Weyman A.E.: Echocardiographic measurement of right ventricular volume. Circulation 1984;69:497-505

65. Starling M.R, Crawford M.H., Sorensen S.G., O'Rourke R.A.: A new two-dimensional echocardiographic technique for evaluating right ventricular size and performance in patients with obstructive lung disease. Circulation 1982;66:612-620

66. Danchin N., Cornette A., Henriquez A., Godenir J.P., Ethevenot G., Polu J.M., Sadoul P.: Two-dimensional echocardiographic assessment of the right ventricle in patients with chronic obstructive lung disease. Chest 1987;92:229-233

67. Linker D.T., Moritz W.E., Pearlman A.S.: A new three-dimensional echocardiographic method of right ventricular volume measurement: in vitro validation. J. Am. Coll. Cardiol. 1986;8:101-106

68. Voelker W., Gruber H.P., Ickrath O., Unterberg R., Karsch K.R.: Determination of right ventricular ejection fraction by thermodilution technique - a comparison to biplane cineventriculography. Intens. Care Med. 1988;14:461-466

69. Marz H.H.: Lungenemphysem und Bronchitis, p. 224. Thieme, Stuttgart. 1963

70. Stevens P.M., Terplan M., Knowles J.H.: Prognosis of cor pulmonale. New. Engl. J. Med. 1963;269:1289-1295

71. Vandenbergh E., Van de Woestijne K.P., Billiet L., Gyselen A.: Evolution et pronostic de la bronchite chronique au stade de la retention de CO_2. Bull Physiopath Resp 1965;1:260-273

72. Blum A.: Die Prognose der chronischen Cor pulmonale. Arch. Kreisl.Forsch. 1965;48:57-68

73. Ouredník A., Jezek V., Baková O.: Pronostic de l'hypertension pulmonaire chez les sujets atteints de bronchite chronique. Bull. Physiopath. Resp. 1968;4:213-224

74. Boushy S.F., Coates E.O.: The prognostic value of pulmonary function tests in emphysema. Am. Rev. Resp. Dis. 1964;90:555-563

75. Cotes J.E.: Prognostic and therapeutic implications of deranged pulmonary function. Proc. Roy. Soc. Med. 1962;55:454-456

76. Mitchell R.S., Weeb N.C., Filley G.F.: Chronic obstructive bronchopulmonary disease. III. Factors influencing prognosis. Am. Rev. Respir. Dis. 1964;89:878-896

77. Pham Q.T., Collombier N., Uffholtz H., Lacoste J., Sadoul P.: Evolution lointaine des hypercapnies chroniques. Bull. Physiopath. Resp. 1965;1:273-290

78. Auchincloss J.H, Gilbert R.: Single-breath diffusing capacity as an aid in evaluation and prognosis of cardiorespiratory disease. Am. Rev. Respir. Dis. 1964;90:28-41

79. Caroll D.: Pulmonary emphysema: report of 26 cases followed to death. Bull. Johns-Hopk. Hosp. 1960;106:154-166

80. Sadoul P., Schrijen F., Uffholtz H., Pham Q.T.: Evolution clinique de 195 pulmonaires chroniques soumis à un cathètèrisme du coeur droit entre 1957 et 1965. Bull. Physiopath. Resp. 1968;4:225-238

81. Weitzenblum E., Hirth C., Ducoloné A. et al: Prognostic value of pulmonary artery pressure in chronic obstructive pulmonary disease. Thorax 1981;36:752-758

82. Massin N., Westphal J.C., Schrijen F., Polu J.M., Sadoul P.: Valeur pronostique du bilan hémodynamique des bronchiteux chroniques. Bull. Eur. Physiopath. Resp. 1979;15:821-837

83. Diener C.F., Burrows B.: Further observations on the course and prognosis of chronic obstructive lung disease. Am. Rev. Resp. Dis. 1975;111:719-724

84. Postma D.S., Burema J., Gimeno F. et al.: Prognosis in severe chronic obstructive disease. Am. Rev. Resp. Dis. 1979;119:357-367

85. Rosenkranz K.A., Drews A., Holling J., Buschmann G.: Zur Hämodynamik des kleinen Kreislauf bei leicht und mittelgradiger Silikose. Beicr. Silik. Forsch. 1965;6:557-564

86. Söderholm B.: The hemodynamics of the lesser circulation in pulmonary tuberculosis. Scand. J. Clin. Lab. Invest. 1957;9 (Suppl 26):1-111

87. Jezek V., Fucík J., Michaljanic A., Jezková L.: The prognostic significance of functional tests in kryptogenic fibrosis alveolitis. Bull. Eur. Physiopath. Resp. 1980;16:711-720

88. Jezek V.: The prognosis and development of pulmonary hypertension in idiopathic diffuse interstitial lung fibrosis. G. Ital. Cardiol. 1984;14 (Suppl 1):39-45

89. Riedel M., Prerovsky I., Stanek V. et al.: Chronic thromboembolic disease. Long-term follow-up. Prog. Resp. Res. 1980;13:134-140

90. Bishop J.M., Cross K.W.: Physiological variables and mortality in patients with various categories of chronic respiratory disease. Bull. Eur. Physiopath. Resp. 1984;20:495-500

91. Voelkel N., Reeves J.T.: Primary pulmonary hypertension. In: Moser K.M. (Ed.), *Pulmonary vascular diseases*, New York, Dekker, 1979; p. 573-628.

92. Mlczoch J.: Evolution of primary pulmonary hypertension. Prog. Resp. Res. 1985;20:176-181

93. Rich S., Levy P.S.: Characteristics of surviving and nonsurviving patients with primary pulmonary hypertension. Am. J. Med. 1984;76:573-578

94. Rozkovec A., Montanez P., Oakley C.M.: Factors that influence the outcome of primary pulmonary hypertension. Br. Heart J. 1986;55:449-458

95. France A.J., Prescott R.J., Biernacki W., Muir A.L., Mac Nee W.: Does right ventricular function predict survival in patients with chronic obstructive lung disease. Thorax 1988;43:621-626

96. Ashutosh K., Dunsky M.: Noninvasive tests for responsiveness of pulmonary hypertension to oxygen. Prediction of survival in patients with chronic obstructive lung disease and cor pulmonale. Chest 1987;92:393-399

97. Galy P., Loire R.: Considérations anatomo-pathologiques sur l'hypertension pulmonaire et les lésions vasculaires au cours de la bronch-pneumopathie chronique dyspnèisante obstructive. Bull. Physiopath. Resp. 1968;4:305-325

98. Bergofsky E.H.: Tissue oxygen delivery and cor pulmonale in chronic obstructive pulmonary disease. New Engl. J. Med. 1983;308:1092-1094

99. Kawakami Y., Kishi F., Yamamoto H., Miyamoto K.: Relation of oxygen delivery, mixed venous oxygenation and pulmonary hemodynamics to prognosis in chronic obstructive pulmonary disease. New Engl. J. Med. 1983;308:1045-1049

100. Harvey R.M.: In: P. Sadoul, (Ed.) *Entretiens de Physiopathologie Respiratoire 1967*, Paris, Gauthier-Villars, 1968; p. 611-612.

101. Kernen J.A., O'Neal R.M., Edwards D.L.: Pulmonary arteriosclerosis and thromboembolism in chronic pulmonary emphysema. Arch. Pathol. 1958;65:471-483

102. Ryan S.F.: Pulmonary embolism and thrombosis in chronic pulmonary emphysema. Am. J. Pathol. 1963;43:767-780

103. Wagenvoort C.A., Heath D., Edwards J.: *The pathology of the pulmonary vasculature*. Thomas, Springfield 1964

104. Macharaoui A., Schött D., Martin W. et al.: Ventrikuläre Rhythmusstörungen bei Cor pulmonale. Einfluss der Sauerstoffbehandlung. Dtsch. Med. Wschr. 1986;111:535-538

Right Ventricular Hypertrophy

2. Differences in the Response of the Right and Left Ventricle to Chronic Hypoxia

B. Ostadal, V. Pelouch, F. Kolar, A. Bass, J. Prochazka, J. Widimsky

Institute of Physiology, Czechoslovak Academy of Sciences, Kardiocentrum, Faculty Hospital Motol and Department of Cardiology, Postgraduate Medical School, Prague, Czechoslovakia

Adaptation to chronic hypoxia is characterized by a variety of functional changes which collectively facilitate oxygen transport from the ambient medium to the cells of the body. All of these changes can be seen at one time or another in the course of hypoxic exposure. Myocardium must maintain adequate contractility in spite of the lowered oxygen tension in the coronary circulation. Such a situation requires adjustment which may protect the heart during conditions which require enhanced work and consequently increased metabolism. Adaptive changes in the chronic hypoxic heart include the effect of increased stress imposed on the right ventricle (RV) by pulmonary hypertension and the actual effect of the reduced partial oxygen pressure; they, therefore, differ in the RV and left ventricular (LV) myocardium.

While it is agreed that disturbances of LV function sooner or later lead to disturbances of RV performance, views of the existence of a reverse mechanism i.e. the possibility of affecting LV function in the presence of a primary disturbance of the RV differ.[1,2,3] Experimental research evolves predominantly in two directions: a) differences between the RV and LV under control conditions and b) right-to-left relationships in pathological situations.

Differences in the Growth of the Right and Left Ventricle under Control Conditions

Important dissimilarities between the two ventricles can be found already in the early phases of ontogenetic development. The difference between the rates of growth of the LV and RV may be interpreted to be the result of the increased work load selectively imposed on the LV. In the fetal lamb during the latter half of gestation, the RV ejects about 60-65% of the combined ventricular output and the

LV ejects only 35-45%, but the end-diastolic pressures in the ventricles, systolic and diastolic pressures in the aorta and diastolic pressures in the aorta and pulmonary artery are equal up to the end of gestation. After lung expansion and clamping of the umbilical cord at birth the peak systolic pressures in the LV and the systemic vascular resistance rise, while the RV pressure, pulmonary artery pressure and pulmonary vascular resistance decrease.[4,5] The increased work load resulting from these circulatory changes is considered to be the stimulus for the more rapid growth of the LV.

The early postnatal heart responds to this stimulus with enlargement, character-ized by an increase in both the number (hyperplasia) and the size (hypertrophy) of its muscle cells, as opposed to the adult myocardium, which responds only by muscle cell hypertrophy. Morphometric studies have shown that during the first 11 days of life in the rat heart, the growth of the LV includes hyperplasia that is not seen in the RV. Average myocyte hypertrophy and binucleation are not significantly different in the RV and LV.[6] The RV/LV ratio decreases after birth and in rats it becomes stabilized only after weaning period.[3] All these results support the statement that ontogenetic differences in the growth response of the RV and LV are not due to genetic expression but to the different work load. Disproportional growth of the RV and LV results in a significantly higher concentration of collagenous proteins in the RV[7,8], since the collagenous fraction develops symmetrically in both ventricles.[9]

There exist other structural, functional and metabolic differences between RV and LV accompanying their different growth; however, the explanation of the functional importance of these changes is often only speculative. A better under-standing of this important question may probably be gained by an investigation of the different reaction of the two ventricles under various pathological conditions.

Differences in the Response of the Right and Left Ventricle to Chronic Hypoxia

Experimental RV hypertrophy, induced by chronic exposure to reduced oxygen tension, results from the striking increase in pulmonary vascular resistance and pulmonary hypertension.[10-12] Much less is known about the effects of chronic hypoxia on the LV. Although the RV is the one exposed to the higher work load, under conditions of chronic hypoxia both ventricles are exposed to the same level of arterial hypoxia. Their growth response depends on the developmental period at which the hypoxic stimulus is applied. In animals exposed to chronic hypoxia in the early phase of postnatal ontogenesis when the muscle cells are still capable of proliferation[13], hypoxia induces enlargement not only of the RV but also a significant, though somewhat lesser enlargement of the LV.[14] Myocardial histoautoradiography in rats exposed to intermittent high altitude on the 30th day of life showed that DNA synthesis in the muscle cell nuclei increases not only in the already enlarged RV, but also in the still unenlarged LV.[15] The muscle cell proliferation may be stimulated either by hypoxia itself or by hypoxia-induced haemodynamic changes.[14,16]

There is a lack of agreement as to whether chronic hypoxia produces LV enlargement in adult animals. Several authors have documented the presence of the LV enlargement both by dissecting the heart and weighing it[10,17,18] and by measuring the myocardial cells in histological sections.[19] These authors exposed rats to chronic hypoxia and found slight LV hypertrophy which was reversed under conditions of continuous normoxia. On the other hand, Recavarren and Arias-Stella[20] and Moret[21] did not observe any LV enlargement. The different degree of hypoxic load as well as the different methodological approach make it impossible to reach an unambiguous conclusion.

We have found in rats that twenty-four exposures to intermittent high altitude hypoxia (IHA, barochamber, stepwise up to 7000 m, 4h/day) did not significantly change RV systolic pressure, but RV hypertrophy could be already seen at this time; the absolute LV weight did not change significantly. When the exposures were prolonged to 8h/day, there was a significant increase in the absolute weight of the RV both after 24 and 60 exposures. The absolute weight of the LV did not change, the relative weight of this part of the myocardium was, however, significantly increased after 60 exposures (Fig. 1).

Our findings demonstrate that RV hypertrophy could be already found in IHA-exposed animals without chronic pulmonary hypertension (24 exposures, 4h/day). Haemodynamic data showed a marked increase of RV systolic pressure during

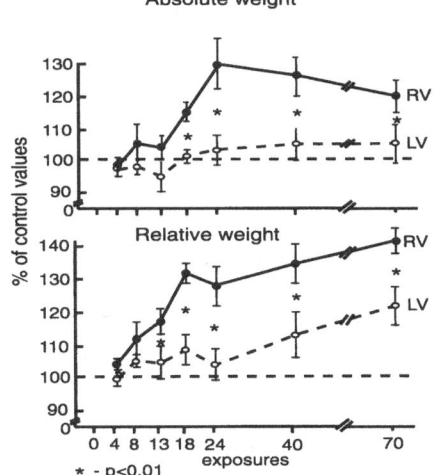

Fig. 1. Absolute and relative weight of the right (RV) and left (LV) ventricle (expressed as % of control values) in rats exposed to intermittent high altitude; x axis - number of exposures (4h/day). Data from 11,22.

inhalation of hypoxic mixture. Accordingly, the findings suggest that RV hypertrophy in our experimental model can be induced by intermittent pulmonary hypertension (present during the stay of the animals in a hypobaric chamber) in relatively short time.[11,22] Our observations were later confirmed by Nattie and Doble[23] who tried to define the threshold value for the development of RV hypertrophy in animals exposed to IHA. They have found that RV enlargement can be found already in animals with 28 exposures to 5500 m when the daily exposure lasted only 2h. These results draw attention to the fact that in patients with pulmonary diseases leading to pulmonary hypertension and cor pulmonale, RV hypertrophy can be present at the stage when pulmonary hypertension is present only intermittently, i.e. during increased pulmonary blood flow (e.g. exercise[24]).

IHA stimulates a proportional increase of myofibrillar and collagenous protein concentration both in the hypertrophic RV and non-hypertrophic LV.[8] Right-to-left differences, characteristic for animals living in a normoxic environment, e.g. higher collagen concentration in the RV, higher concentration of myofibrillar proteins in the LV, did not change. Collagen is increased in all experimental models of cardiac hypertrophy except in that of nutritional anaemia.[25]

Hypoxia is well known to be a specific stimulus for fibroblastic activity and it seems to be responsible for the proliferation of collagenous stroma in both parts of the heart of hypoxic rats.

IHA caused significant rise in circulating blood volume; this was due to increased haematocrit. The myocardial perfusion in the LV and RV markedly increased. The relative increase in the RV was greater: whereas RV perfusion (measured by ^{86}RbC1) in the controls represented 74,6% of the LV, in rats exposed to IHA it approaches values of the LV perfusion[26] (Fig. 2).

No substantial changes in the capillary supply to the LV were found in animals adapted to high altitude.[27] The values of cardiac output were significantly higher in IHA exposed rats as compared with controls (31.75 ± 2.29 ml/100 g body weight vs. 21.59 ± 1.25 ml/100 g).[26] Intermittent low pressure exposures seems to be more severe stress in comparison with permanent hypoxia simulating an altitude of 3500m[28], where the cardiac output was not elevated. The basic cause for higher relative organ flow and increased cardiac output is probably due to tissue hypoxia with a greater blood flow demand. The actual mechanism is not known but may be influenced by higher sympathetic activity.

Chronic hypoxia may stimulate favourable myocardial adaptation as well as imposing a stress, the magnitude of which depends upon the intensity of hypoxia. We have observed IHA-induced acute focal necrotic lesions, localized predominantly in the RV[11] with the development of disseminated myofibrosis and/or chronic aneurysm of the RV wall. It is interesting to note, that such primarily affected myocardium is significantly more resistant to acute hypoxia or necrogenic stimulus.[11,29,36]

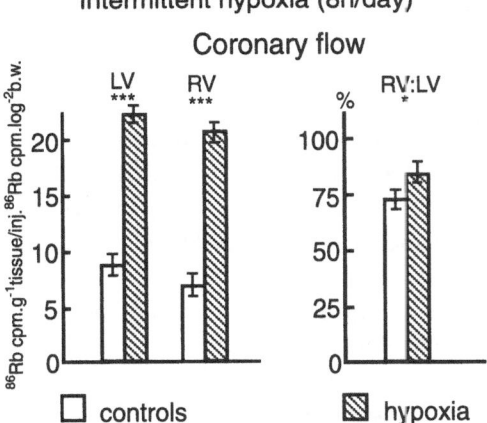

Fig. 2. Right (RV) and left (LV) ventricular perfusion in rats exposed to intermittent high altitude (24 exposures, 8h/day, 5 days a week); *** - p<0.001; * - p<0.02. Data from 26.

Chronic Hypoxia-Induced Changes in Energy Metabolism in the Right and Left Ventricular Myocardium

The metabolic response of the myocardium to altitude hypoxia depends on the intensity and duration of the hypoxic stimulus. In acute (a few hours' or days') exposure to a natural altitude (3454 m - the Jungfraujoch), significant changes occurred in metabolite levels in the heart of the laboratory rat; creatine phosphate, ATP and glycogen reserves fell very low, whereas the lactate and pyruvate concentration and the lactate/pyruvate ratio rose, i.e. glycolysis was activated.[30] Gold and Costello[31] found a decrease in the dehydrogenases of the tricarboxylic acid cycle in rats exposed for seven days to a simulated altitude of 7500 m. During a moderately long period (4-12 weeks) on the Junfraujoch[30], creatine phosphatase and ATP showed a gradual return to normal, but glycogen levels were still low. During a long stay (up to 50 weeks), the values in question returned to normal, evidently as a sign of metabolic adaptation of the myocardium.

In this connection, we were interested in ascertaining how acclimatization to IHA would affect the activity of certain enzymes of energy metabolism. We studied enzyme activities associated with different ways of obtaining energy - with the phosphorylation of glucose, with anaerobic glycolysis, with aerobic metabolism and with the oxidation of fatty acids - in both the hypertrophic RV and in non-hypertrophied LV.[32]

In the control animals, no significant differences were found between the given enzyme activities in the RV and LV. After 24 and 72 four-hour exposures to IHA, we observed significant (15-30%) elevation of hexokinase activity (HK, glucose phosphorylation) in both ventricles; an analogous trend was observed in the case of lactate dehydrogenase (LDH). The other activities of enzymes associated with anaerobic glycolysis (triosephosphate dehydrogenase - TPDH, glucose-6-phosphate dehydrogenase - GPDH) and of enzymes associated with aerobic metabolism (malate dehydrogenase - MDH, citrate synthase - CS) did not alter significantly. On the other hand, hydroxyacyl-CoA-dehydrogenase (HOADH) activity decreased in both ventricles although the decrease was not significant until after the 72nd exposure (Table I).

Prolongation of the daily exposure time from 4 to 8h did not lead to further intensification of the above changes.

Our results show that the capacity for utilizing glucose (HK) and the capacity for synthesizing and degrading lactate (LDH) increase significantly in both ventricles

Table I. Activity of enzymes of energy metabolism (as percentages of the control values ± SEM) in the right (RV) and left (LV) ventricle; intermittent hypoxia, 4 h daily, 24 and 72 exposures. * Difference from the controls statistically significant ($p<0.01$)

	24 exposures		72 exposures	
	RV (n=6)	LV (n=6)	RV (n=6)	LV (n=6)
LDH	125.4±16.6	113.9±18.5	111.7±17.9	132.7±19.7
TPDH	104.0 ± 5.0	110.9± 5.4	114.2±10.3	102.5± 6.0
GPDH	96.5±14.0	116.5±21.0	84.2 ± 4.3	83.5± 8.5
HK	130.3± 7.8*	118.1± 8.8*	117.1± 7.2*	115.0± 7.2*
MDH	106.9±17.6	101.4±18.8	111.3±20.5	108.3±20.7
CS	97.3±12.4	87.1±16.6	91.2±11.6	83.8± 7.7
HOADH	85.9±16.4	83.6±20.0	68.8±10.5*	67.9±10.0*

during acclimatization to IHA. Conversely, there is a significant drop in the ability to break down fatty acids (HOADH). Thus increased oxidation of glucose and lactate evidently occurs at the expense of fatty acids. These changes appeared only after 24 four-hour exposures; prolongation of the hypoxic stimulus did not lead to any further marked shifts.

All the above changes in the enzyme profile were found in the hypertrophic RV but also in the non-hypertrophied LV.

In the literature relatively numerous studies can be found dealing with metabolic aspects of the effect of chronic altitude hypoxia on the myocardium. Some authors concentrated on the dynamics of changes in metabolites and reserve substances (glycogen, CrP, ATP, etc)[30,33], while others studied lipid accumulation[34] or individual enzyme activities. For instance, Tenney and Ou[35] observed an increase in succinate dehydrogenase activity in rats. Only Barrie and Harris[36] used a large set of enzymes of energy metabolism in guinea pigs exposed permanently to a high altitude (5000 m, 28 days).

They showed that metabolic changes induced in the myocardium by acclimatization to altitude hypoxia were the resultant of several different phenomena, which undoubtedly include the effect of a lowered food intake (both the RV and LV), the specific effect of the increased stress imposed on the RV by pulmonary hypertension and the actual metabolic effect of the reduced partial oxygen pressure (again both ventricles). To differentiate the effect of a diminished food intake, the above authors used a second control group with a limited food intake.

Anorexia was associated with a decrease in glycogen phosphorylase and hexokinase activity. RV hypertrophy was accompanied by an increase in glycogen phosphorylase, phosphoglucomutase, hexokinase, glucose-phosphate isomerase, triosophosphate dehydrogenase and phosphoglycerate kinase activity. A reduced food intake and hypertrophy both led to an increase in the proportion of LDH M subunits.

Lastly, chronic hypoxia itself (evaluated from changes in the LV) was characterized by an increase in hexokinase, triosophosphate dehydrogenase and phosphoglycerate kinase activity.

However, as Barrie and Harris[36] admitted, since the LV was also slightly hypertrophied, the possibility that the increase observed in the given enzyme activities may also be associated with enlargement of this compartment of the heart cannot be ruled out.

Evidently, adaptation to chronic hypoxia significantly influences the metabolism of the myocardium; this effect has not yet been unequivocally elucidated, however. Differentiation of the direct effect of hypoxia from the effect of functional hypertrophy and of other extracardial factors presents great problems and the whole situation is complicated by large differences in the methods and in the choice of the experimental animals.

The difference between the effect of acclimatization and genetically coded changes in a population living permanently at high altitudes is equally unclear. In general, it can be claimed that the number of serious studies in this sphere is relatively small and that each of them explains a situation defined by the chosen type of hypoxia, the experimental animals and the spectrum of the metabolic parameters studied.

As distinct from the cited available studies using continuous hypoxia, our results can be regarded as the first contribution to the study of metabolic responses of the myocardium to IHA of varying duration.

Chronic Hypoxia-Induced Cardiopulmonary Changes in Young Animals

Whereas relatively numerous studies can be found dealing with the effect of chronic hypoxia on the adult cardiopulmonary system, much less is known about the response of the immature organism. We have, therefore, compared the effect of chronic hypoxia simulated in barochamber (8h per day, 5 days a week, stepwise up to 7000 m, total of 24 exposures) on some functional and metabolic parameters in rats acclimatized from the 4th day or the 12th week of postnatal life.[37,38]

IHA induced a significant increase in the total heart weight and the RV weight in both age groups; the absolute LV weight remained unchanged. The heart growth response, expressed in relative units, was significantly higher in animals acclimatized to IHA from birth. IHA leads to marked chronic pulmonary hypertension; the pressure rise (as judged from the RV systolic pressure) was significantly higher in adults (by 62.8%) when compared with young animals (by 45.5%). Furthermore, RV weight increased linearly with a rise of pulmonary blood pressure in animals exposed to IHA from the 4th day of life (r=0.72); this relationship was, however, very loose in adult rats (r=0.16).

Smith et al.[39] reported that young rats exposed to chronic hypobaric hypoxia showed a lower RV hypertrophy than in adult animals. In this study, however, the young group was not acclimatized before the 21st day of life; furthermore, no haemodynamic measurements were carried out. Rabinowitch et al.[40] compared cardiopulmonary changes in rats exposed to permanent hypoxia (corresponding to an altitude of 5500 m), starting either from the 9th day of life or in adults. They found that young animals respond to hypoxia by slightly higher pulmonary hypertension and RV enlargement than adult rats; the differences were not statistically significant. The degree of structural remodelling of pulmonary vascular bed was, however, significantly higher in younger animals. It is obvious that the literature data referring to the ontogenetic development of the cardiopulmonary system in chronic hypoxia are scarce and often contradictory. Different results and conclusions may be due to methodological variability (different models of hypoxia (permanent vs. intermittent), the length and intensity of hypoxic exposure, anaesthesia) as well as the species, strain and maturity of experimental animals.

Our finding that in young animals a lower degree of pulmonary hypertension was connected with greater RV enlargement supports the opinion that the ventricular growth response to chronic hypoxia differs during development. The stimulus may be both the decrease of PO_2 as well as the secondary influence of altered haemodynamics. The close correlation between both parameters in young hypoxic rats may thus be the consequence of the higher "reactivity" of developing heart.

Acclimatization to IHA significantly changes the protein profile of the rat cardiac muscle, predominantly in the RV.[41] In young animals, IHA delayed the transformation of isomyosin V3 to V1, which normally occurs during ontogeny.

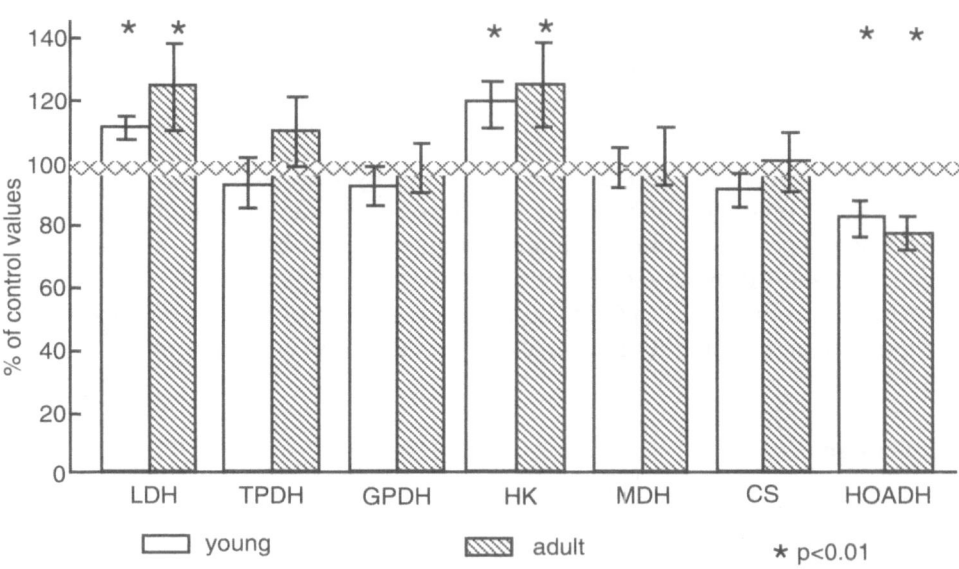

Fig. 3. Enzymes of the energy supplying metabolism (expressed as % of control values) in rats exposed to intermittent high altitude from the 4th day (young) or 12th week (adult) of postnatal life. Data from 37,38.

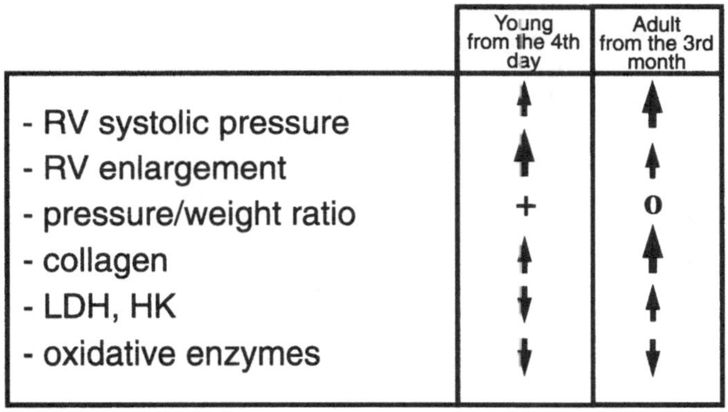

	Young from the 4th day	Adult from the 3rd month
- RV systolic pressure	↑	↑
- RV enlargement	↑	↑
- pressure/weight ratio	+	0
- collagen	↑	↑
- LDH, HK	↓	↑
- oxidative enzymes	↓	↓

Fig. 4. Comparison of the response of the cardiopulmonary system of young and adult rats to chronic hypoxia. Data from 37,38.

22

This results in an increased proportion of isomyosin V3, as it does in adult hypoxic rats; such shifts are connected with decreased ATPase activity of the myosin molecule.[42] Moreover, IHA significantly stimulates the formation of collagen III in adult animals. In young rats IHA increased both types of collagen, but the elevation of collagen III was significantly higher (120:160%); the functional significance of structural changes of collagen is, however, unclear. The chronic hypoxia-induced changes in energy metabolism described above were comparable in both age groups (Figs. 3, 4).

It may be concluded, that the effect of chronic hypoxia, simulated in barochamber, induced functional and metabolic changes in the cardiopulmonary system in both young and adult animals. Significant ontogenetic differences may be consequence of the different sensitivity to hypoxic stress; nevertheless, ontogenetic differences in other factors, participating in the regulation of circulatory homeostasis, cell growth and proliferation have also to be taken into consideration.

References

1. Jezek V: Vzajemny vztah mezi funkci prave a leve srdecni komory. Cs. fysiol. 1978;3:278
2. Widimsky J: *Pulmonale Hypertonie*. Georg Thieme Verlag, Stuttgart, New York, 1981
3. Ostadal B., Urbanova D., Ressl J., et al.: Changes in the right and left ventricles in rats exposed to intermittent high altitude hypoxia. Cor. Vasa 1981; 23:111
4. Rudolph A.M.: Distribution and regulation of blood flow in the fetal and neonatal lamb. Circ. Res. 1985; 57:811
5. Peterson C.J., Whitman V., Watson P.A., et al.: Mechanism of differential growth of heart ventricles in newborn pigs. Circ. Res. 1989; 64:360
6. Anversa P., Olivetti G., Loud A.V.: Morphometric study of early postnatal development in the left and right ventricular myocardium of the rat. Circ. Res. 1980; 46:495
7. Oken D.E., Boucek R.J.: Quantitation of collagen in human myocardium. Circ. Res. 1957;5:357
8. Ostadal B., Mirejovska E., Hurych J., et al: Effect of intermittent high altitude hypoxia on the synthesis of collagenous and non-collagenous proteins of the right and left ventricular myocardium. Cardiovasc. Res. 1978; 12:303
9. Caspari P.G., Gibson K., Harris P.: Collagen and myocardium. A study of their normal development and relationship in the rabbit. Cardiovasc. Res. 1975; 9:187
10. Abraham A.S., Kay J.M., Cole R.B., et al: Haemodynamic and pathological study of the effect of chronic hypoxia and subsequent recovery of the heart and pulmonary vasculature of the rat. Cardiovasc. Res. 1971;5:95
11. Widimsky J., Urbanova D., Ressl J., et al: Effect of intermittent altitude hypoxia on the myocardium and lesser circulation in the rat. Cardiovasc. Res. 1973;7:798
12. Fishman A.P.: Hypoxia on the pulmonary circulation. How and where it acts. Circ. Res. 1976; 30:221
13. Zak R.: Development and proliferative capacity of cardiac muscle cells. Circ. Res. 1974; 35: suppl II, 134
14. Hollenberg M., Honbo N., Samorodin A.J.: Effects of hypoxia on cardiac growth in neonatal rats. Amer. J. Physiol. 1976; 231:1445

15. Wachtlova M., Mares V., Ostadal B.: DNA-synthesis in the ventricular myocardium of young rats exposed to intermittent high altitude (IHA) hypoxia. An autoradiographic study. Virchows Arch. B. Cell. Path. 1977; 24:335

16. Arefyeva A.M., Mares V., Ostadal B., et al: A cytophotometric and karyometric study of the cardiac muscle cells of young rats exposed to intermittent high altitude hypoxia. Physiol. bohemoslov. 1985; 34:94

17. Cook C., Barer G.R., Shaw J.W., et al: Growth of the heart and lungs in normal and hypoxic rodents. J. Anat. 1980; 107:384

18. Sizemore D.A., McIntyre T.W., Van Liere E.J., et al: Regression of altitude produced cardiac hypertrophy. J. Appl. Physiol. 1973; 35:518

19. Clark D.R., Smith P.: Capillary density and muscle fibre size in the hearts of rats subjected to simulated high altitude. Cardiovasc. Res. 1978; 12:578

20. Recavarren S., Arias-Stella J.: Right ventricular hypertrophy in people born and living at high altitudes. Brit. Heart J. 1964; 26:806

21. Moret P.R.: Hypoxia and the heart. In: Bourne G.H (Ed), *Hearts and heart-like organs*. New York, Academic Press, 1980; vol 2, pp 333-387

22. Ostadal B., Widimsky J.: *Intermittent hypoxia and cardiopulmonary system*. Academia, Prague 1985

23. Nattie E.E., Doble E.A.: Threshold of intermittent hypoxia-induced right ventricular hypertrophy in the rat. Resp. Physiol. 1984; 56:353

24. Widimsky J., Dejdar R., Kubat K., et al: The growth of the muscular and collagenous parts of the heart in various forms of cardiomegaly. J. Physiol. 1969; 200:285

26. Kasalicky J., Ressl J., Urbanova D., et al: Relative organ blood flow in rats exposed to intermittent high altitude hypoxia. Pflügers Arch. 1977; 368:111

27. Rakusan K., Turek Z., Kreuzer F.: Myocardial capillaries in guinea pigs native to high altitude (Junin, Peru, 4,105 m). Pflügers Arch. 1981;391:22

28. Turek Z., Turek-Maischeider R.A., Claessens R.A., et al: Coronary blood flow in rats native to simulated high altitude and in rats exposed to it later in life. Pflügers Arch. 1975;355:49

29. Poupa O., Krofta K., Prochazka J., et al: Acclimatization to simulated high altitude and acute cardiac necrosis. Fed. Proc. 1966; 25:1242

30. Moret P.R.: Myocardial metabolism: Acute and chronic adaptation to hypoxia. Medicine Sport Sci. 1985; 19:48

31. Gold A.J., Costello L.C.: Effects of altitude and semistarvation on heart mitochondrial function. Amer. J. Physiol. 1974; 227:1336

32. Bass A., Ostadal B., Prochazka J., et al: Intermittent high altitude-induced changes in energy metabolism in the rat myocardium and their reversibility. Physiol. bohemoslov. 1989; 38:155

33. Ostadal B., Prochazka J., Pelouch V., et al: Comparison of cardiopulmonary responses of male and female rats to intermittent high altitude hypoxia. Physiol. bohemoslov. 1984; 33:129

34. Gloster J., Hasleton P.S., Harris P., et al: Effect of chronic hypoxia and diet on the weight and lipid content of viscera in the guinea pig. Environm. Physiol. Biochem. 1974;4:251

35. Tenney S.N., Ou L.C: Some tissue factors in acclimation to high altitude. In: Hegnauer, *Biomedicine of high terrestrial elevations*. USARIEM, 1969

36. Barrie S.E., Harris P.: Effect of chronic hypoxia and dietary restriction on myocardial enzyme activities. Amer. J. Physiol. 1976; 231:1308

37. Kolar F., Ostadal B., Prochazka J., et al: Comparison of cardiopulmonary response to intermittent high altitude hypoxia in young and adult rats. Respiration 1989; 56: 57

38. Ostadal B., Kolar F., Pelouch V., et al: The effect of chronic hypoxia on the developing cardiopulmonary system. Biomed. Biochim. Acta 1989; 48: S58

24

39. Smith P., Moosavi H., Winson M., et al: The influence of age and sex on the response of the right ventricle, pulmonary vasculature and carotid bodies to hypoxia in rats. J. Pathol. 1974; 112:11
40. Rabinowitch M., Gamble J.W., Miettinen O.S., et al: Age and sex influence on pulmonary hypertension of chronic hypoxia and on recovery. Amer. J. Physiol. 1981; 240:H62
41. Pelouch V., Ostadal B., Prochazka J., et al: Effect of high altitude on the protein composition of the right ventricular myocardium. Progr. Resp. Res. 1985; 20:41
42. Pelouch V., Ostadal B., Prochazka J.: Changes of contractile and collagenous proteins induced by chronic hypoxia in myocardium during postnatal development of rat. Biomed. Biochem. Acta 1987;46:707.

3. Function of the Hypertrophic Right and Left Ventricles in Experimental Conditions

R. Cihak[1], F. Kolar[2], V. Pelouch[2], J. Prochazka[2], B. Ostadal[2], J. Widimsky[1]

1. Department of Cardiology, Postgraduate Medical and Pharmaceutical Institute, Czechoslovak Academy of Sciences, Kardiocentrum, Faculty Hospital Motol and Department of Cardiology, Postgraduate Medical Scool, Prague, Czechoslovakia
2. Institute of Physiology, Czechoslovak Academy of Sciences, Kardiocentrum, Faculty Hospital Motol and Department of Cardiology, Postgraduate Medical Scool, Prague, Czechoslovakia

Introduction

The heart responds to a chronically increased load by an important adaptive mechanism, myocardial hypertrophy. The condition involves comprehensive and dynamic transformation of the heart at the level of organ, cells, and subcellular structures. However, the adaptive process, in addition to its positive aspects, includes adverse changes that may be associated with functional impairment and the development of cardiac failure.

It is known from clinical practice that the prognosis of patients with left ventricular (LV) hypertrophy is poor[1] and, even though hard evidence regarding the prognostic value of right ventricular (RV) hypertrophy is unavailable yet, failure of the hypertrophic right ventricle is also a frequent finding.[2]

To study the properties of cardiac muscle in various phases of development of hypertrophy, a number of models are employed.[3,4] While the main differences between these models consist in the type, intensity and duration of the hypertrophy-inducing load, they may also differ in the biological aspects, i.e., the species, age and sex of the experimental animal. Depending on these variables, the stage of hypertrophy at which the heart is investigated, also varies.[5,6]

The functional properties are evaluated in the isolated papillary muscle as well as "in vitro" and "in vivo" function of the heart using various parameters of systolic and diastolic function, both at rest and during exercise. As a rule, only one ventricle is assessed, with the data obtained in these studies applied generally to the entire hypertrophic myocardium. Very heterogeneous results can be encountered in the literature, with the function of the hypertrophic heart alternately reported as normal, increased and decreased.[7,8] Numerous experimental and clinical studies have demonstrated that, once the cause of cardiac hypertrophy had been eliminated, regression occurs.[9,10] However, it is still poorly understood whether the decrease in cardiac mass is associated with normalization of its structural as well as functional properties,[11] with only few data available in the literature.

Our study, using three models of cardiac hypertrophy, was designed to compare some functional and structural properties accompanying the development of cardiac hypertrophy and its regression. Both ventricles were assessed.

Materials and Methods

Our experimental animals were adult male Wistar rats aged 3 months $\pm$ 10 days assigned to the following groups:

Isoprenaline. A total of 44 rats were given isoprenaline (Isoprenaline Spofa) at a dose of 0.25 mg. kg^{-1} s.c. for 10 days. A control group of 36 animals was administered saline.

Thyroxine. Forty-four rats were given thyroxine (L-thyroxine Serva) at a dose of 0.30 mg.kg^{-1} s.c. for 10 days. A control group of 40 control animals received the same volume of saline.

High-altitude hypoxia. A group of 44 rats was exposed to intermittent high-altitude hypoxia in a hypobaric chamber. The initial simulated altitude rose from 2000 m to 7000 m during 13 exposures (8 hrs/day, 5 days a week), the total number of exposures was 24.[12, 13] When outside the chamber, the animals were kept under normoxic conditions, as were 36 control rats.

The experimental and control animals were divided into two groups, one investigated in the phase of hypertrophy 24 hours after the last exposure (dose), the other one evaluated in the phase of regression of hypertrophy 35 days after load discontinuation.

The function of both ventricles was assessed "in vivo" in animals under general anaesthesia (Thiopental Spofa, 50 mg.kg^{-1} i.p.). Both groups (experimental and control) were again split into two subgroups, with LV function studied in one, and RV function in the other.

In our study, the LV testing load was acute ligature of the ascending aorta.[14] After connecting the animals to artificial ventilation (Zimmermann ventilation pump), sternotomy was performed to insert a probe with an inner diameter of 0.8 mm into the left ventricle transmurally via the apex. Pressure changes from the ventricle were transmitted via the probe to an induction pressure recorder (Hewlett Packard 1280), amplified to be digitalized, using a (Sapi 1, Tesla) microcomputer, and tape recorded. The studied parameters, derived from the pressure curve, included peak pressure increase rate (dP/dt_{max}). Our definition of functional reserve was the difference between dP/dt_{max} before and after load, i.e., before and after aorta ligation

(Fig. 1a). A similar technique was employed to assess RV function; a probe was introduced transmurally into the RV to monitor the response to acute pulmonary artery ligation (Fig. 1b).

Following function measurement, the heart was removed from the thorax and dissected into the left and right ventricles and the septum, with each part weighed separately.[15] The percentage of dry weight was also determined in all specimens.

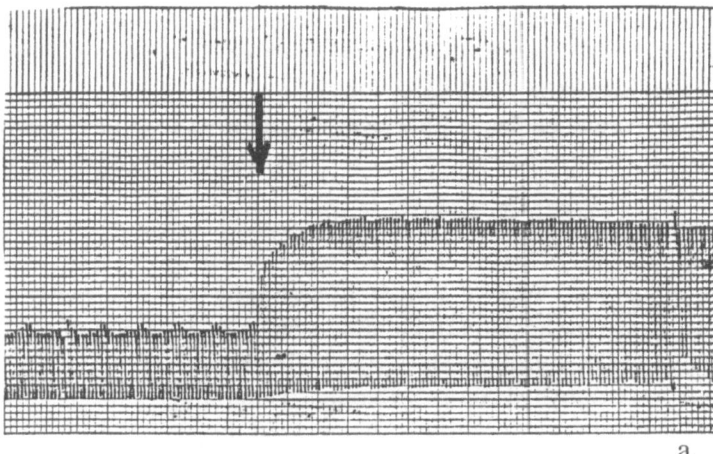

a

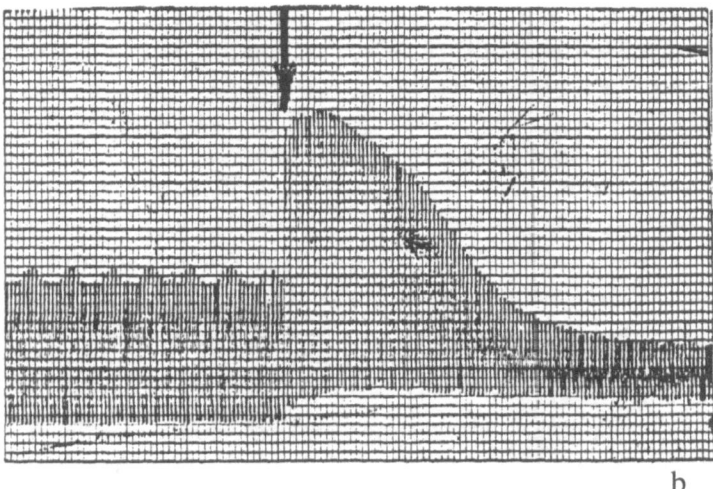

b

Fig. 1. The left (a) and right (b) ventricular pressure before and after acute aorta (a) and pulmonary artery (b) clamping.

Structural impairment was suggested by changes in the amount of collagen. Samples of dried tissue from the left and right ventricles were used to determine the concentration and content of hydroxyproline, i.e., the amino acid present almost exclusively in collagen. Hydroxyproline levels were assessed using the conventional method according to Stegeman.[16] Weighed samples were hydrolysed by hydrochloric acid (HC1) and, following neutralization with sodium hydroxide (NaOH), chloramine T, perchloric acid ($HClO_4$) and dimethylaminobenzaldehyde (PDAB) were added gradually to the hydrolysate. Hydroxyproline content was determined in samples, treated as described, by photometry at a wavelength of 550 nm (Spekol 10 photometer, Carl Zeiss Jena).

Results were evaluated statistically using Student's t-test for two independent groups.

Results

A mild to moderate degree of cardiac hypertrophy was induced in all models (Table I). Titration of the hormone dose allowed us to produce a comparable degree of hypertrophy in both thyroxine and isoprenaline models. While LV weight rose by 20%, RV hypertrophy was more pronounced attaining a value as high as 30%. Exposure to intermittent high-altitude hypoxia led to isolated 50% RV hypertrophy, with total heart weight increasing by 14%. The fact that no significant decrease in the body weight of experimental animals was documented suggested a similar magnitude of relative cardiac hypertrophy.

Five weeks after discontinuation of the hypertrophy-inducing load, heart weight did not differ in any of the models from that of controls, with a slightly increased LV weight persisting in the isoprenaline group only (Tab. I). The ratio of dry/wet weight of the heart did not change throughout the experiment. The amount of dry weight in the left and right ventricles ranged within 21-23%.

Just as in the experimental groups (in the phases of hypertrophy and regression), LV and RV function was evaluated also in the control groups. This design enabled us to compare results of a total of six control groups for each ventricle. Variability of results was low, with the resting values of dP/dt_{max} of the right ventricle being within the range of 1250-1550 mmHg s^{-1}, and 5000-5600 mmHg s^{-1} in the left ventricle. The dP/dt_{max} increased after acute load to approximately double the resting values (Figs. 2-4).

In the high-altitude model, the resting values of dP/dt_{max} of the RV were increased. The higher mass of contractile musculature led to higher values also after the acute load (pulmonary artery ligation - Fig. 4). Surprisingly, a very similar pattern was observed also in the RV of the thyroxine group (Fig. 2). In the isoprenaline group, the values of dP/dt_{max} at rest and after acute load did not differ from those of controls (Fig. 3). RV functional reserve did not differ from that of

Table I. Weight characteristics of animal groups. n-number of animals, BW-body weight, HW-heart weight, RV-right ventricle, LV-left ventricle. Values are expressed as mean ± SEM; * - $p < 0.05$; ** - $p < 0.01$ vs. controls

Thyroxine	n	BW (g)	HW (mg)	RV (mg)	LV (mg)
controls	14	418±10	952±26 **	201±6 **	547±17 **
hypertrophy	14	393±11	1167±35 **	268±9 **	658±23 **
controls	14	468± 9	959±20	211±7	543±18
regression	14	470±13	1002±21	218±7	562±21
Isoprenaline					
controls	12	352±10	832±25 **	178±7 **	466±12 **
hypertrophy	14	339± 7	1037±19 **	246±6 **	565±17 **
controls	12	445±12	933±17	212±8	516±13
regression	14	444±14	983±21	213±7	558±12 *
High Altitude					
controls	16	453±11	926±23	206± 9	509±18
hypertrophy	18	421±12	1060±25 *	305±11 **	526±16
controls	16	492±15	982±32	201± 7	564±24
regression	18	480±15	1011±27	216± 8	568±21

controls in any of our models. The resting values of dP/dt $_{max}$ of the hypertrophic LV were normal in the thyroxine model, and mildly increased in the isoprenaline model. The findings obtained after aorta clamping were quite different: while the functional reserve of the thyroxine group was markedly increased, it was decreased in the isoprenaline group (Figs 2,3). Function of the non-hypertrophic LV of the high-altitude group was normal (Fig. 4).

Whereas LV and RV function completely normalized with regression of hypertrophy in most of the models, functional impairment persisted in the LV of the isoprenaline model (Figs 2-4).

The development of hypertrophy after isoprenaline was associated with a considerable increase in collagen concentration, but in the LV only (Fig. 6). By contrast, collagen concentration in both ventricles was normal in the thyroxine model (Fig. 5). This shows the content of myocardial collagen depends on the model of hypertrophy, and there may be a difference also between LV and RV.

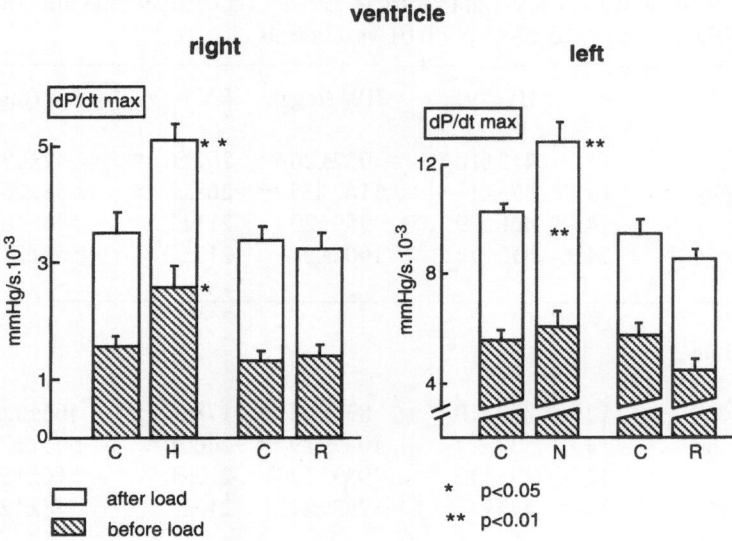

THYROXINE

ventricle

right · left

Fig. 2. Experimental cardiac hypertrophy after thyroxine administration. The function of the right and left ventricle before and after acute load, i.e. pulmonary artery and aorta clamping. (C-controls, H-group with hypertrophy, R-group after regression of hypertrophy).

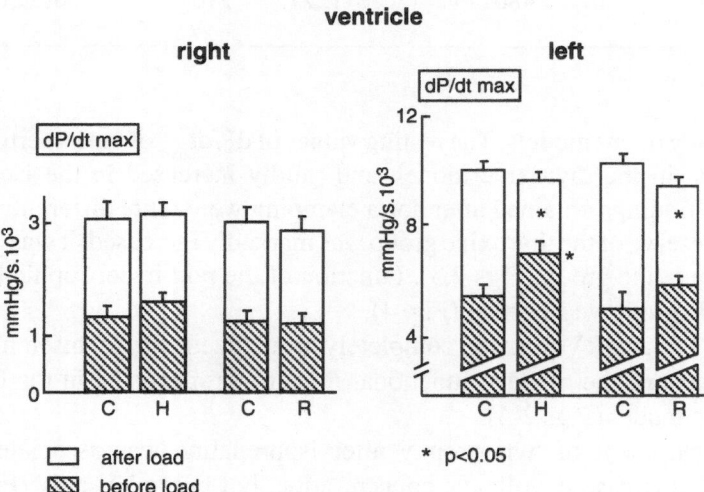

ISOPRENALINE

ventricle

right · left

Fig. 3. Experimental cardiac hypertrophy after isoprenaline administration. The function of the right and left ventricle before and after acute load, i.e. pulmonary artery and aorta clamping. (C-controls, H-group with hypertrophy, R-group after regression of hypertrophy).

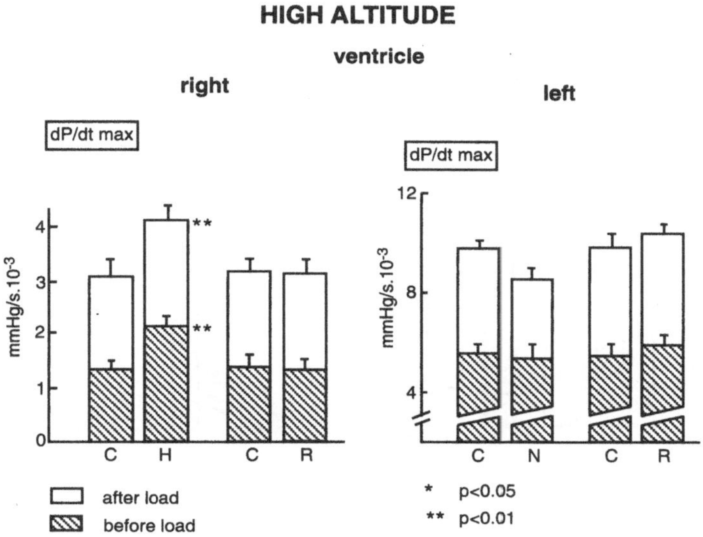

HIGH ALTITUDE

ventricle

right   left

Fig.4. Experimental cardiac hypertrophy after exposure to intermittent high altitude hypoxia. The function of the right and left ventricle before and after acute load, i.e. pulmonary artery and aorta clamping.
(C-controls, H-group with hypertrophy, R-group after regression of hypertrophy).

The mild increase in collagen, documented also in the LV following high-altitude hypoxia, indicates changes occur also in the ventricle not exposed to the primary load (Fig. 7).

The increased collagen concentration in the LV of animals after high-altitude hypoxia and, especially, after isoprenaline, persisted as long as 5 weeks after load discontinuation. At that time also an increase in the RV manifested itself, an observation suggesting the structural myocardial impairment was not reversible. By contrast, no difference was again demonstrated in the thyroxine model compared with the right and left ventricles of controls. Collagen concentration was found to rise with age - a minor increase was observed just after 5 weeks in both ventricles of all control groups (Figs. 5-7).

Discussion

The design of our study involves the same periods of thyroxine and isoprenaline administration, and the same degree of LV and RV hypertrophy. This enables us to compare two models of cardiac hypertrophy with completely different myocardial impairment while minimizing all other variable factors. Hypertrophy of both ventricles was compared with a model of isolated RV hypertrophy in a group exposed to high-altitude hypoxia.

32

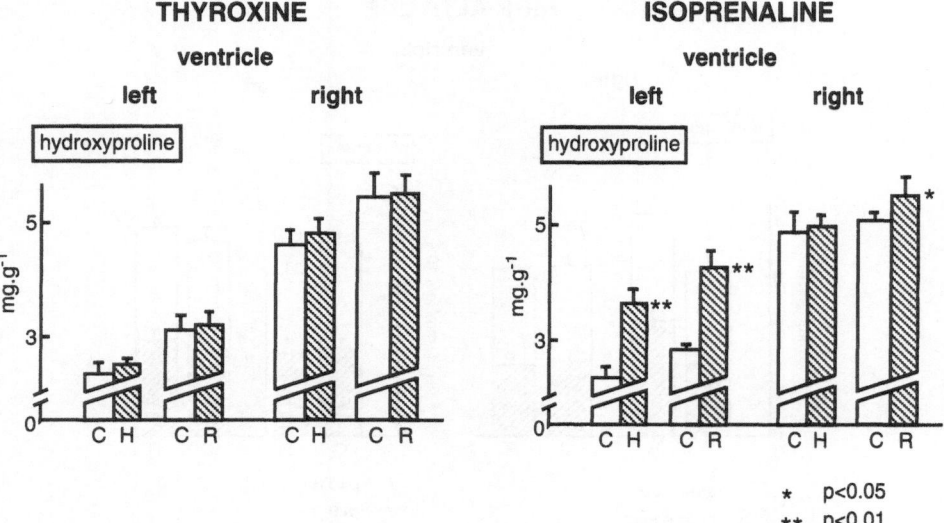

THYROXINE

ventricle

left   right

ISOPRENALINE

ventricle

left   right

* p<0.05
** p<0.01

Fig. 5. Experimental cardiac hypertrophy after thyroxine administration. The hydroxyproline concentration in the left and right ventricle. (C-controls, H-group with hypertrophy, R-group after regression of hypertrophy).

Fig. 6. Experimental cardiac hypertrophy after isoprenaline administration. The hydroxyproline concentration in the left and right ventricle. (C-controls, H-group with hypertrophy, R-group after regression of hypertrophy).

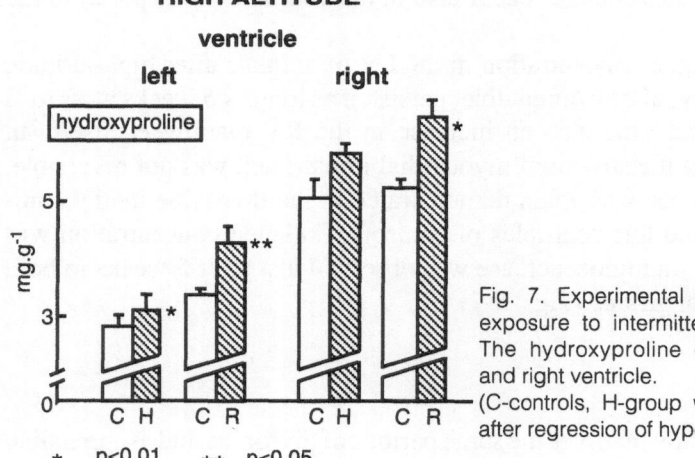

HIGH ALTITUDE

ventricle

left   right

* p<0.01   ** p<0.05

Fig. 7. Experimental cardiac hypertrophy after exposure to intermittent high altitude hypoxia. The hydroxyproline concentration in the left and right ventricle. (C-controls, H-group with hypertrophy, R-group after regression of hypertrophy).

In all of our models, the function of the hypertrophic RV was increased or normal. The values of dP/dt$_{max}$ in the high-altitude hypoxia model were elevated. A surprising finding was that of a very similar pattern also in the RV following thyroxine administration; our tentative explanation of the pulmonary hypertension observed in this model is hyperkinetic circulation.[17] Compared with the findings made in the RV, those in the two models of LV hypertrophy were different. While the LV functional reserve in the thyroxine model was markedly increased, it was decreased in the isoprenaline model. They are, in fact, two opposite models. When referring to the thyroxine model, some authors speak of so-called "physiological" hypertrophy; the effect of isoprenaline resembles, in contrast, pathological pressure overload.[18]

Experimental data about the function of the hypertrophic heart are very heterogeneous, just as the models of hypertrophy are. [7,8] The results correlate directly with the duration and degree of stress and the magnitude of hypertrophy, as demonstrated by Spann in his review.[19] A mild stenosis of the pulmonary artery in the cat produces 36% RV hypertrophy while papillary muscle function is normal. A more marked stenosis and 90% hypertrophy are accompanied by decreased contractility; a 90% stenosis causes 140% hypertrophy with *in vivo* signs of heart failure. A similar correlation was reported to exist in the left ventricle. Functional deterioration is thus related to the attainment of a "critical weight" of the ventricle and, hence, pronounced hypertrophy.[20]

Only models of acute pressure load often show rapid myocardial impairment and a decrease in function.[21,22] Our results indicate the different findings need not be associated only with the degree of hypertrophy and the rate of onset of overload. Completely different functional properties, just as hypertrophic left and right ventricles in the same model, may also be found in models with a comparable degree of hypertrophy.

The quantity of myocardial connective tissue also depends on the model of hypertrophy. While collagen concentration remains unchanged after some types of load, it does rise in most models.[23] Age and sex of the experimental animals also play a role.[24,25]

In our study, no change in myocardial collagen concentration was documented in either ventricle in the thyroxine model throughout the experiment. By contrast, a marked increase, however in the LV only, was seen in the isoprenaline model. Connective tissue growth is associated with the direct stimulating effect of isoprenaline on collagen synthesis but, also, with the development of myocardial necrotic lesions that can be noted even after low doses.[26] An explanation of the difference between left and right ventricles could be the lower RV oxygen uptake and higher coronary reserve and, hence, a smaller extent of necrosis. The isolated effect of isoprenaline on increasing collagen production in the LV cannot be dismissed either.

However, this latter possibility is less probable, since it was just the RV in which isoprenaline caused more marked hypertrophy. Besides, the stimulus of collagen synthesis acts more often on the heart as a whole. This is confirmed also by the non-hypertrophic LV.[12,13] Unlike the LV of the isoprenaline model, there was no functional impairment. The fibrosis, however, was mild and it is quite possible that, to demonstrate deteriorated function using our method, more marked fibrosis is necessary.

Five weeks after chronic load discontinuation, regression of hypertrophy and RV and LV function normalization were seen in most models. Collagen content remained unaltered and, as a result of regression of myocyte hypertrophy, collagen concentration rose markedly also in the RV of the high-altitude hypoxia model after isoprenaline. Regression of myocardial hypertrophy is not associated with the decrease in collagen content.[27,29]

Spontaneous regression of collagen has been reported very rarely, with speculation about a possible effect on the amount of connective tissue by some drugs such as Ca^+ antagonists or angiotensin-converting enzyme inhibitors.[30,31] Yet another plausible explanation is that a substantially longer period of time is necessary to detect collagen regression.[32]

No agreement regarding cardiac function following regression of hypertrophy has been reached yet. Most papers report a normal function after regression of cardiac hypertrophy of various causes.[21,22,33,34] They are often unable to distinguish changes due to a decrease in afterload from those caused by regression of hypertrophy.[11] At the same time, it should be remembered that functional impairment may be manifested in some of the measured parameters, and in some exercise tests only.[35,36] In our experiments, RV as well as LV function after regression of hypertrophy was quite normal, both at rest and after acute load. Only in the isoprenaline model, with no complete regression of LV hypertrophy attained, and a markedly increased collagen concentration, did functional impairment persist.

Functional impairment of the heart is due to changes in the structural and biochemical composition of the myocardium.

The most important of these changes include increased interstitial tissue concentration. The increase leads to depletion of musculature available for contraction, decreases myocardial compliance and increases the barrier to oxygen-metabolite exchange processes that, when combined with the decreased coronary reserve and increased oxygen uptake, may contribute to a further rise in fibrosis.[37-39]

The changes involve not only the total amount of myocardial collagen but, also, representation of the individual types of collagen and their distribution in various tissue structures.[29,40] The significance of collagen heterogeneity is not clear, but it is possible that substitution of one type by another affects also the mechanical properties of the heart.[41] The pathophysiological mechanism of development of heart failure is doubtless very complex, with a number of other factors possibly involved to various extents.[42] A role is played by the limitation of the magnitude of hypertrophy and, hence, insufficient adaptation to increasing load.[43]

However, it is probable that it is just the irreversible rise in collagen concentration which is one of the key mechanisms of onset of functional impairment and its persistence even after the cause of cardiac hypertrophy has been eliminated.

The results of our study show that the development of hypertrophy in individual experimental models is associated with a variety of functional and structural changes: hearts with a comparable degree of hypertrophy may be found to have completely different properties.

The implication is that, when assessing cardiac hypertrophy, one cannot apply exclusively the weight criterion since it is not necessarily a reliable marker of the stage in cardiac hypertrophy. Even though the left and right ventricles respond similarly to a chronic load, it has been shown that accurate assessment of the development of changes requires parallel follow-up of both. This is indicated by the findings obtained in models of hypertrophy involving the whole heart, a condition in which the same changes need not be present in both ventricles. Findings made in one ventricle cannot serve as a basis for the assessment of changes in the properties of the other ventricle. Moreover, the high-altitude hypoxia model suggests that the non-hypertrophic ventricle, not directly affected by the load, also responds in a way.

The initial stage of RV and LV hypertrophy is invariably regarded as a positive adaptive change. The increased amount of contractile elements allows the hypertrophic heart to raise its function. Elimination of the cause of hypertrophy results in its spontaneous regression. A decrease in the amount of the musculature is associated with functional normalization; the left as well as right ventricle is usually normal following regression of mild hypertrophy. Depending on the character, intensity and duration of stress, however, the adverse consequences of the adaptive process gradually prevail. This is followed by the development of structural myocardial impairment accompanied by functional impairment. Elimination of the stress need not lead to complete regression of hypertrophy: the increased collagen concentration persists as does functional impairment. It can be concluded that the changes associated with the development of hypertrophy are not invariably reversible.

References

1. Kannel W.B., Sorlie P.: Left ventricular hypertrophy in hypertension: Prognostic and pathogenetic implications. The Framingham Study. In: Strauer B.E. (Ed.) *The heart in hypertension*, Berlin, Springer Verlag 1981; 223-242

2. Fishman A.P.: Cor pulmonale: General Aspects. In: Fishman A.P. (Ed.) *Pulmonary diseases and disorders*, New York, McGraw Hill Book Co. 1980; 397-409

3. Hamrell B.B., Alpert N.R.: Cellular basis of the mechanical properities of hypertrophied myocardium. In: Fozzard H.A.(Ed.) *The heart and cardiovascular system*, New York, Raven Press 1986;1507-1524

4. Mann D.L., Spann J.F., Cooper G.: Basic mechanism and models in cardiac hypertrophy. Mod. Concepts Cardiovasc. Dis. 1988; 57:7-11

36

5. Meerson F.Z.: The myocardium in hyperfunction, hypertrophy and heart failure. Circ. Res., 25 (suppl. II): 1969;163.

6. Zak R.: Overview of the growth process. In: Zak R. (Ed.) *Growth of the heart in health and disease*, New York, Raven Press 1984; 1-24

7. Skelton C.L., Sonnenblick E.H.: Heterogeneity of contractile function in cardiac hypertrophy. Circ. Res., 1974, 34-35 (suppl. II): 83-91

8. Sonnenblick E.H., Strobeck J.E., Capasso J.M., Factor S.M.: Ventricular hypertrophy: models and methods. In: Tarazi R.C., Dunbar J.B. (Ed.) *Cardiac hypertrophy in hypertension, Perspectives in cardiovascular research* Vol. 8, New York, Raven Press 1983; 13-20

9. Beznak M., Korecky B., Thomas G.: Regression of cardiac hypertrophies of various origin. Can. J. Physiol., Pharmacol. 1969; 47:579-586

10. Ressl J., Urbanova D., Widimsky J., Ostadal B., Pelouch V., Prochazka J.: Reversibility of pulmonary hypertension and right ventricular hypertrophy induced by intermittent high altitude hypoxia in rats. Respiration 1974; 31: 38-46

11. Tarazi R.C., Frohlich E.D.: Is reversal of cardiac hypertrophy a desirable goal of antihypertensive therapy? Circulation 1987; 75 (suppl. I): 113-117

12. Widimsky J., Urbanova D., Ressl J., Ostadal B., Pelouch V., Prochazka J.: Effect of intermittent altitude hypoxia on the myocardium and lesser circulation in the rat. Cardiovasc. Res. 1973;7:798-805

13. Ostadal B., Widimsky J.: Intermittent hypoxia and cardiopulmonary system. Academia, Praha 1985; 92

14. Goodkind M.J.: Left ventricular myocardial contractile response to aortic constriction in the hyperthyroid guinea pig. Circ. Res. 1968; 22:605-614

15. Fulton R.M., Hutchinson E.C., Jones A.M.: Ventricular weight in cardiac hypertrophy. Brit. Heart J. 1952;14: 413-420

16. Stegeman H.: Mikrobestimung von Hydroxyprolin mit Chloramin T und p-dimetylaminobenzaldehyd. Hoppe Seylers Zeitschrift für Physiologische Chemie 1958; 311:41-45

17. Zierhut W., Zimmer H.G.: Effect of triiodothyronine on hemodynamic and metabolic parameters of the right ventricle in the rat. J. Mol. Cell. Cardiol. 1987; 19 (suppl. III): 112

18. Wikman-Coffelt J., Parmley W.W., Mason D.T.: The cardiac hypertrophy process. Analyses of factors determining pathological vs. physiological development. Circ. Res. 1979; 45:697-707

19. Spann J.F.: Functional changes in pathologic hypertrophy. In: Zak R.(Ed.) *Growth of the heart in health and disease.* Raven Press, New York 1984; 421-466

20. Messerli F.H., Schmieder R.: Left ventricular hypertrophy a cardiovascular risk factor in essential hypertension. Drugs 1986; 31 (suppl.4): 192-201

21. Cooper G., Satava R.M., Harrison C.E., Cileman H.V.: Normal myocardial function and energetics after reversing pressure overload hypertrophy. Am. J. Physiol. 1974; 226: H1158-1165

22. Capasso J.M., Strobeck J.E., Malhotra A., Scheuer S., Sonnenblick E.H.: Contractile behaviour of rat myocardium after reversal of hypertensive hypertrophy. Am J. Physiol. 1982; 242:H882-887

23. Bartosova D., Chvapil M., Kopecky B., Poupa O., Rakusan M., Turek Z., Visek M.: The growth of the muscular and collagenous parts of the rat heart in various forms of cardiomegaly. J. Physiol. 1969; 200:285-295

24. Wachtlova M., Ostadal B., Mares V.: Thyroxine induced cardiomegaly in rats of different age. Physiol. Bohemoslov. 1985; 34:385-394

25. Williams J.F., Potter R.D., Mathew B.: Time dependency of myocardial mechanical performance after pulmonary artery banding in cats. In: Alpert N.R.(Ed.) *Myocardial hypertrophy and failure,*

Perspectives in cardiovascular research Vol. 7, New York, Raven Press 1983; 271-280

26. Collins P., Billings C.G., Barer G.R., Doly J.J., Jolly A.: Quantitation of isoprenaline induced changes in the ventricular myocardium. Cardiovasc. Res. 1975; 9:797-806

27. Cutilletta A.F., Dowell T., Rudnik M., Arcilla R.P., Zak R.: Regression of myocardial hypertrophy: J. Mol. Cell. Cardiol. 1975; 7: 767-780

28. Sen S., Tarazi R.C., Bumpus F.M.: Reversal of cardiac hypertrophy in renal hypertensive rats: medical vs. surgical therapy. Am. J. Physiol. 1981; 240: H 408-412

29. Pelouch V., Ostadal B., Prochazka J., Urbanova D., Widimsky J.: Effect of high altitude hypoxia on the protein composition of the right ventricular myocardium. Progr. Resp. Res. 1985; 20:41-48

30. Zähringer J.: Biochemische Veränderungen bei Herzmuskelhypertrophieregression. Z. Kardiol. 1985; 74 (suppl.7): 119-126

31. Motz W., Strauer B.E.: Left ventricular function and collagen content after regression of hypertensive hypertrophy. Hypertension 1989; 13:43-50

32. Krayenbuehl H.P., Ritter M., Hess O., Schneider J., Hall G., Turina M.: Left ventricular structure in aortic stenosis early and late after valve replacement. Europ. Heart J. 1987; 8 (suppl. 2): 101

33. Wisenbaugh T., Allen P., Cooper G., Connor W.N., Mezaros L. et al.: Hypertrophy without contractile dysfunction after reversal of pressure overload in the cat. Am. J. Physiol. 1984; 247: H146-154

34. Strauer B.E., Motz W., Bürger S.: Myocardial and metabolic consequences of development and regression of cardiac hypertrophy in chronic heart disease. In: Alpert N.R. (Ed.) *Myocardial hypertrophy and failure. Perspectives in cardiovascular research* Vol. 7, New York, Raven Press 1983; 633-672

35. Speech M.M., Ferrario C.M., Tarazi R.C.: Cardiac pumping ability following reversal of cardiac hypertrophy and hypertension in spontaneously hypertensive rats. Hypertension 1980; 2: 75-82

36. Saragoca M.A., Tarazi R.C.: Left ventricular hypertrophy in rats with renovascular hypertension. (Alterations in cardiac function and adrenergic responses). Hypertension 1981; 3 (suppl. II): 171-176

37. Bing O.H., Sen S., Conrad C.H., Brooke W.W.: Myocardial function, structure, and collagen in the spontaneously hypertensive rats: progression from compensated hypertrophy to haemodynamic impairment. Eur. Heart J. 1984; 5 (suppl. F): 45-52

38. Bishop S.P., Hittinger L., Shannon R.P., Vatner S.F.: Myocardial fibrosis in cardiac hypertrophy with and without congestive heart failure. Circulation 1988; 78 (suppl. II): 604

39. Holubarsch Ch., Holubarsch T., Jacob R., Medugorac I., Thiedeman K.: Passive elastic properties of myocardium in different models and stages of hypertrophy: A study comparing mechanical, chemical, and morphometric parameters. In: N.R. Alpert (Ed.) *Myocardial hypertrophy and failure, Perspectives in cardiovascular research Vol. 7*, New York , Raven Press, 1983; 323-336

40. Weber K.T., Clark W.A., Janicki J.S., Shroff S.G.: Physiologic vs. pathologic hypertrophy and the pressure overload myocardium. J. Cardiovasc. Pharmacol. 1987; 10 (suppl.6): 37-49

41. Weber K.T.: Cardiac interstitium in health and disease: the fibrillar collagen network. J.Am. Coll. Cardiol. 1989; 13: 1637-1652

42. Jacob R., Vogt M., Rupp H.: Pathophysiological mechanism in cardiac insufficiency induced by chronic pressure - an attempt to analyze specific factors in animal experiment. Basic. Res. Cardiol. 1986; 81 (suppl. 1): 203-216

43. Taylor S.H.: Influence of drug therapy on myocardial hypertrophy in left ventricular failure. J. Cardiovasc. Pharmacol. 1987; 10.Suppl.6:141-147

4. Ontogenetic Development of the Protein Composition of the Right and Left Ventricular Myocardium

V. Pelouch, M. Milerova, B. Ostadal, J. Prochazka

Institute of Physiology, Czechoslovak Academy of Science, Kardiocentrum, Faculty Hospital Motol and Department of Cardiology, Postgraduate Medical School, Prague, Czechoslovakia

Introduction

The postnatal development of the cardiac muscle represents a broad spectrum of morphological, biochemical and physiological changes; ultimately it is a set of cellular and subcellular adaptations to new physiological conditions. Cardiac development in the prenatal period is characterized by a spontaneous but declining cell proliferation,[1] accumulation of different enzymes occasioned by increased aerobic metabolism,[2,3] increase in the number of myocytes and mitochondria, and maturation of various cell organelles.[4] It is well established that postnatal development of the cardiac muscle occurs primarily by cellular hypertrophy due to enhanced protein synthesis.[5]

The impulse for the higher synthesis is initiated in part by the work load imposed on the heart.[6,7] The limited proliferative capabilities and rapid structural and functional maturation of ventricular myocytes in early postnatal development are well documented[8] but the exact temporal sequence of these events remains still to be clearly established. Two major differences between young and adult myocardium have been described: the diameter of the fetal cell is smaller than that of the adult one and the proportion of noncontractile mass (e.g. nuclei, mitochondria and membrane surfaces) relative to the number of myofibrils is significantly higher than in the adult.[3]

This article is concerned with quantitative and qualitative developmental changes in individual proteinaceous structures. Since the early phase of postnatal myocardial development includes also the maturation of membranous myocardial formations (sarcoplasmic reticulum, sarcolemma) which participate not only in the maintenance of the intracellular and extracellular milieu[9] but, above all, in the transport of calcium, we studied also these structures. Membrane integrity depends on glycolytically generated ATP[10] and the study concentrated therefore also on changes in glycogen which is the main substrate for glycolytic processes.

Materials and Methods

Male Wistar rats of different ages were used in the study. All male rats born on the same day were pooled and then assigned to dams randomly to make eight animals per litter. This litter size was maintained until 28 days after birth and the animals then were placed in groups of 4 rats in cage and given food (diet DOS 2B) and water ad libitum until the experiment.

Tissue preparation

Rats were first weighed and then killed. The hearts were divided into three parts (right ventricle, left ventricle and septum) by the methods of Fulton,[12] recommended by the expert committee of WHO[13] and individual parts were weighed separately.

Fractionation of cardiac muscle

Right and left ventricle (freed of vessels) were washed with deionized water, cut into small pieces and briefly homogenized. The samples of both chambers were treated consecutively with different buffers (Fig.1) to obtain the fraction of sarcoplasmic, contractile and collagenous proteins.[14] The protein was determined according to Lowry.[15]

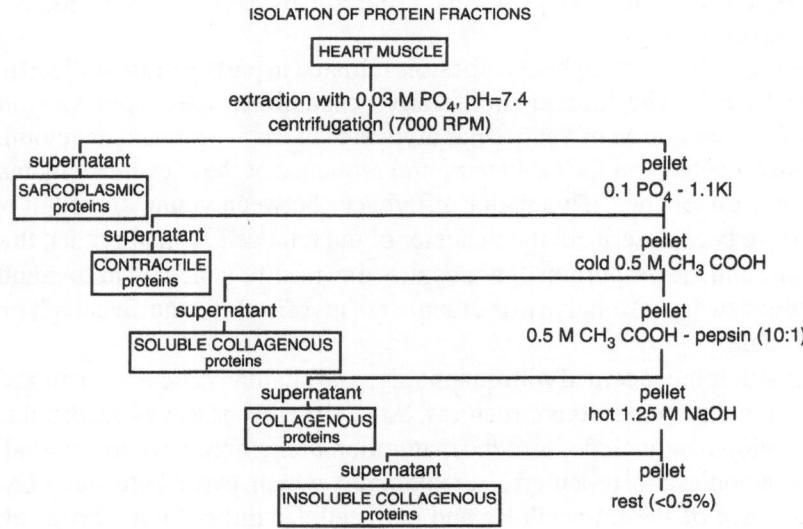

Fig. 1. Scheme of isolation of different protein fractions.

ATPase activity of cardiac myosin
Myosin was isolated in parallel from the right and left ventricles[16], the calcium ATPase activity of myosin[11] was measured at 25°C in 20 mM TRIS, 0.6 M KCl, 5.5 mM ATP in the presence of 10 mM CaCl (pH=7.5).

Hydroxyproline
The concentration of the amino acid hydroxyproline in the collagenous protein fraction was estimated.[17]

Ca uptake by sarcoplasmic reticulum
Sarcoplasmic reticulum vesicles were isolated and calcium uptake was measured by Ca selective electrodes (Oregon USA) in a medium containing 0.1 M KCl, 6 mM $MgCl_2$, 5 mM azide and 10 mM TRIS HCl (pH=7.0) containing also 5 mM potassium oxalate in 20 mM TRIS HCl buffer.[18]

Free radical membrane scavengers
Cardiac tissue was homogenized using the Polytron in a mixture of 5% NaEDTA-ethanol. The samples were homogenized once more in n-hexane. The hexane phase was used for measuring the vit. E and active pool of scavengers by the diphenylpicrylhydrazyl test at 508 nm. Hexane extracts were then treated with 1.4% NaOH and used for determining the total antiradical activity.[19]

Cardiac glycogen
After hydrolysis of the cardiac tissue (20 min. at 100° C-30%KOH), glycogen was precipitated from the supernatant by ethanol. The concentration of glycogen was estimated after acid hydrolysis.[32]

Statistical differences
All results were expressed as means ± SEM. The significance of differences between the groups was tested by Student's test. The differences were considered statistically significant at $p<0.05$ or less.

Results

Quantitative changes in proteinaceous structures

Protein profiling
The transition from the juvenile to the adult circulation is characterized by increasing circulatory demands; both the volume load that acts on both ventricles and the pressure load acting predominantly on the left ventricle increased. The outcome of the adaptative developmental process in the perinatal period is thus a

42

faster growth of the left ventricle, the right/left ratio decreasing in parallel (Fig. 2). During the postnatal development of both cardiac compartments the protein composition of the right and left ventricle changes in a characteristic manner. The concentration of contractile proteins (Fig. 3) in the two compartments is the same in newborn rats. Subsequently the concentration in both compartments rises, the increase being faster in the left ventricle.

Hence a significant right/left difference is observed already on the day 15 after birth. In adulthood the difference disappears but the concentration in the left ventricle remains higher. Substantially smaller differences were detected in the fraction of sarcoplasmic proteins (Fig. 4). In newborn rats the concentration is again the same, during the postnatal development phase of the right ventricle the concentration of this fraction drops transiently and gives rise to a right/left difference which disappears in adulthood. The myocardial development is further accompanied by increase in the concentration of collagenous proteins (Fig. 5 - the sum of soluble and insoluble fraction of collagenous proteins) and by the elevation of the concentration of hydroxyproline, an amino acid typical for collagen (Fig. 6). Already on the day 15 after birth the concentration of collagen is significantly higher in the right ventricle. This higher concentration of collagen (measured by means of hydroxyproline) in the right ventricle persists even in adulthood (Fig. 6). Although the concentration of all collagenous proteins during myocardial development increases significantly, we were unable to detect any significant right/left differences (Fig. 5).

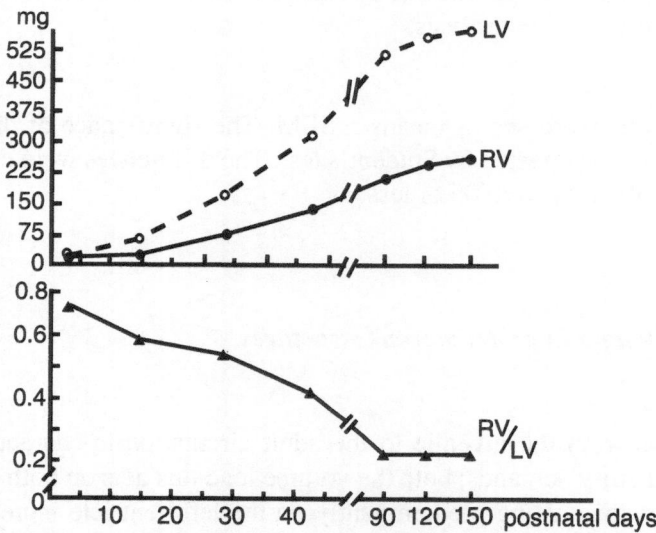

Fig. 2. The right (RV) and left (LV) ventricular weight and the right to left ratio (RV/LV).

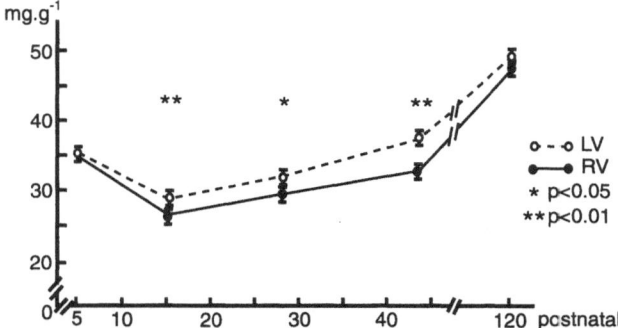

Fig. 3. Concentration of contractile proteins in the right (RV) and left (LV) ventricles. Asterisks mean significant differences between both ventricles. Data are expressed as mg of proteins per g of wet weight.

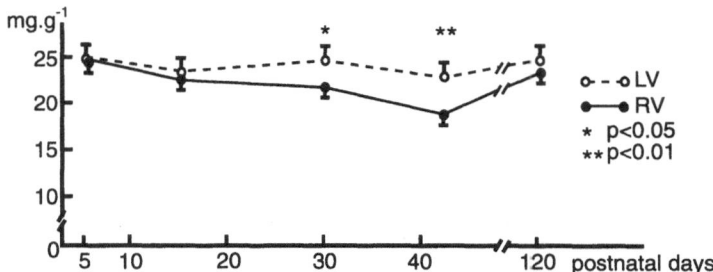

Fig. 4. Concentration of sarcoplasmic proteins in the right (RV) and left (LV) ventricles. For details see Fig. 3.

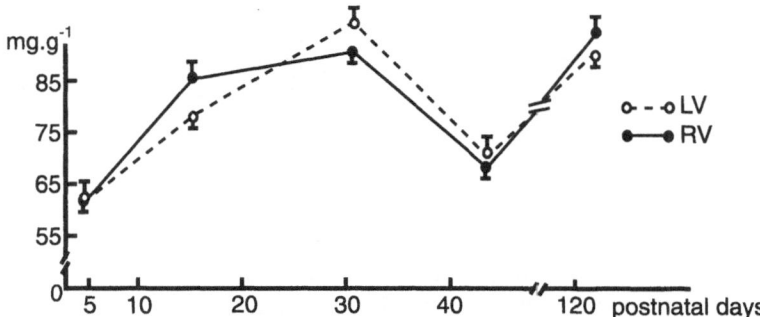

Fig. 5. Concentration of collagenous proteins (sum of soluble and insoluble fractions in the right (RV) and left (LV) ventricles. For details see Fig. 3.

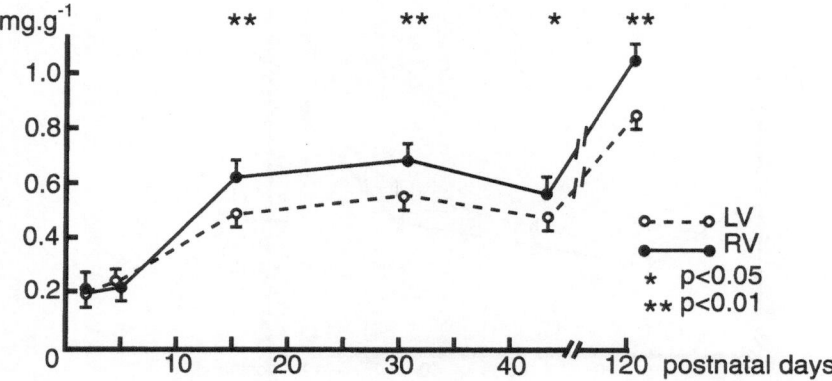

Fig. 6. Concentration of hydroxyproline in the right (RV) and left (LV) ventricles. For details see Fig. 3.

Qualitative changes in proteinaceous structures

1. The ATPase activity of myosin

Newborn rats exhibit a low enzymatic activity of myosin in both myocardial ventricles. In the postnatal period the ATPase activity increases significantly; the increase is higher in the right ventricle, giving rise to a significant right/left difference which persists till sexual maturity. We found that in adult animals the ATPase activity in both compartments decreases and the right/left difference disappears (Fig. 7).

2. Ca uptake by sarcoplasmic reticulum

During the first two weeks of postnatal life the uptake of calcium ions in the left ventricle increases significantly (Fig. 8) and attains 75% of the adult values on the day 15 after birth. The time course in the right ventricle does not differ from that in the left ventricle (data not shown).

3. Alteration of free radical scavenger level in the myocardial membrane

During cardiac development both the qualitative and quantitative composition of lipophilic scavengers changes. In newborn animals the concentration of tocopherol in both compartments is relatively high and then drops by about a half. Between the 15th and the 60th postnatal day it does not change and in adulthood it increases in both compartments. No significant right/left differences were observed throughout the whole ontogenetical development (Fig. 9). The total pool of membrane-bound hydrophobic scavengers is high in newborn animals and declines significantly already on the 15th postnatal day. This decline persists till adulthood when the values are about 25% relative to those found in newborns. As in tocopherol, no

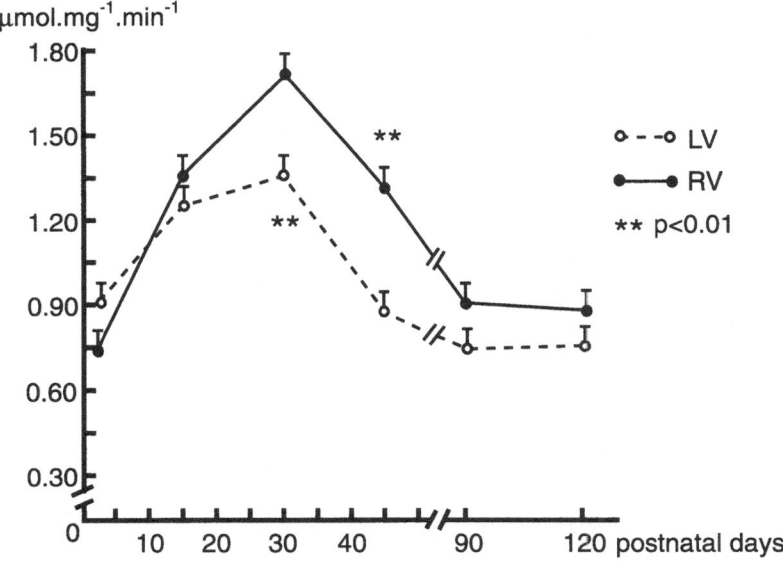

Fig. 7. Ca-ATPase activity of myosin isolated from the right (RV) and left (LV) ventricles. For details see Fig. 3. Values expressed as μmol of inorganic phosphate per min per mg of proteins.

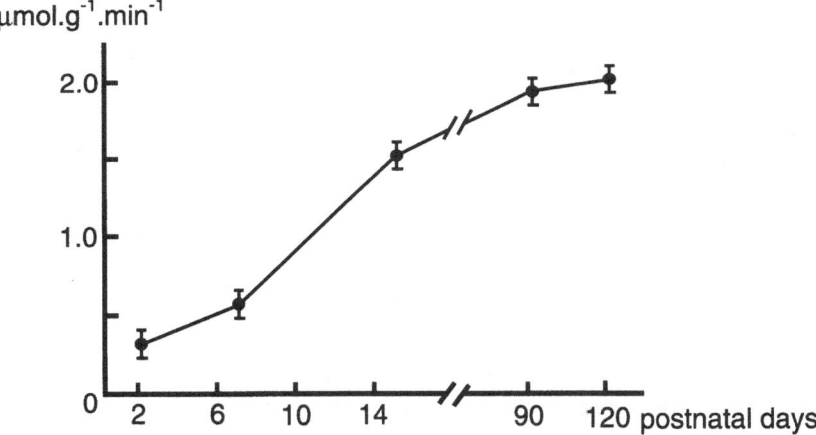

Fig. 8. Ca²⁺ uptake of sarcoplasmic reticulum vesicles isolated from the left ventricle. Values as μmol of calcium per min per gram of wet weight.

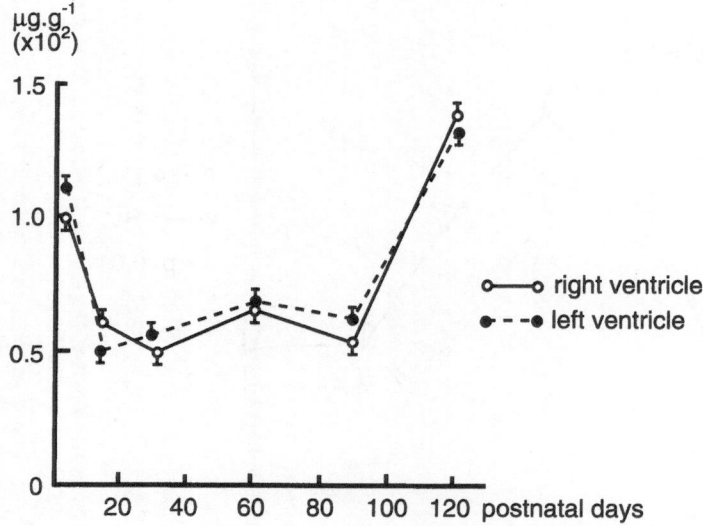

Fig. 9. Concentration of tocopherol (vit. E) in cardiac membranes isolated from the right (RV) and left (LV) ventricles. Values expressed as μg per gram of wet weight (x 100).

significant right/left differences were found. In contrast the relative proportion of active scavengers (represented mostly by tocopherol) in the total pool increases in the course of myocardial development. In newborns it is about 15%, in adulthood around 60% (Fig. 10).

4. Changes in glycogen

The concentration of glycogen in both ventricles decreases during ontogenetical development. In newborn animals the concentration is 6 times higher than in adults (Fig.11). This decrease was observed in both ventricles and it takes place predominantly during the first postnatal month.

Discussion

The growth of the cardiac muscle in the postnatal period reflects predominantly increased cellular protein synthesis initiated by the work load imposed on the heart.[6,20]

The mechanism by which an altered work load is transformed into a growth response is the contraction of the cardiac muscle per se; the work performed by the myocardium stimulates both the total cell protein content and protein synthesis.[5] In the course of the first three postnatal months the rats in our experimental set exhibited a 14-fold increase in the right ventricular weight, and a massive 28-fold increase in left ventricular weight. Although actual weight differences between the

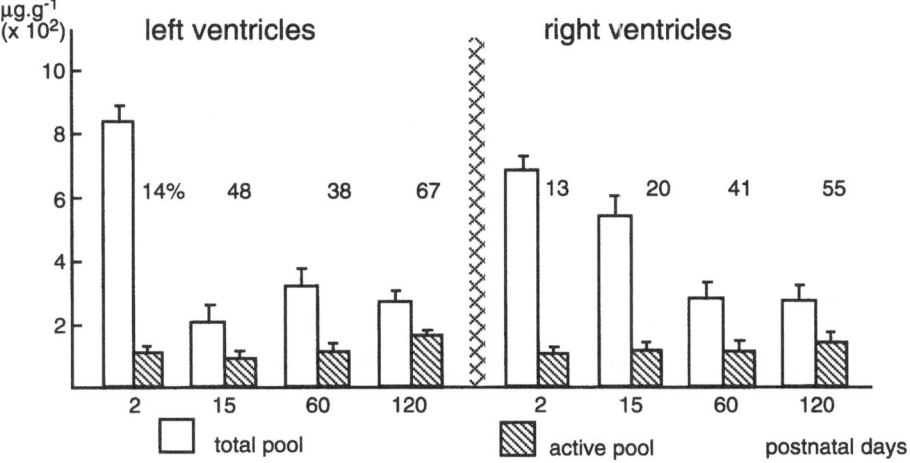

Fig. 10. Concentration of hydrophobic scavengers in membranes isolated from the right and left ventricles. Data are expressed as μg unit of vit. E per gram of wet weight.

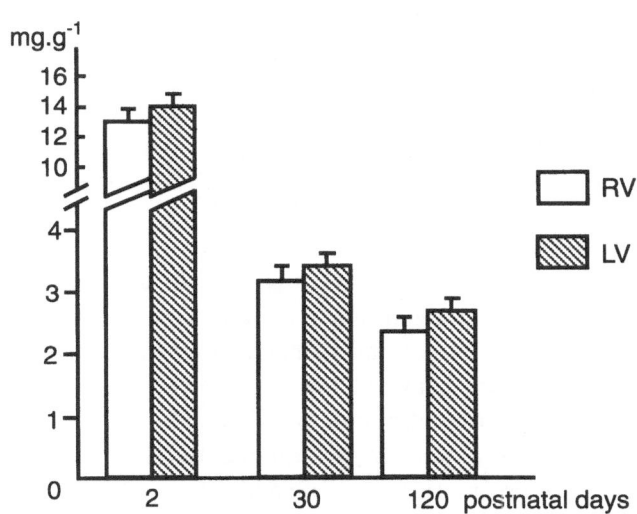

Fig. 11. Concentration of cardiac glycogen in the right (RV) and left (LV) ventricles. Values are expressed as mg of glycogen per gram of wet weight.

right and the left ventricle depend on a number of factors (animal species, strain, nutrition regime, etc) the growth of the left ventricle in the early postnatal period is always faster.

The myocardium is composed of material formed by muscular and interstitial compartments whose relative proportion and physical arrangement determine the myocardial function.[21] We studied the qualitative and quantitative changes in proteinaceous structures of both ventricles. A stepwise fractionation of the tissue[14] yielded three basic fractions: *sarcoplasmic* proteins containing predominantly proteins responsible for metabolic reactions - glycolytic enzymes, Krebs cycle enzymes, etc; *contractile* proteins responsible for cardiac muscle contractility; and *collagenous* proteins that represent a supporting structure for myocytes.

Contractile proteins represent a set of proteins which transform the chemical energy of ATP in the myofibril to the mechanical work of the myocardium. They consist of two major components (myosin and actin), and include also regulatory proteins and some minor protein components (modulatory proteins). The function and structure of individual components have been the subject of numerous reviews[22,23], the most copious data being available on myosin. Developmental changes of heart myosin were described in rabbits and rats[11,24,25,26], less conspicuous changes occur in sheep, mice, pigs and humans.[23,27,29,30]

The changes are associated with both the light and the heavy chains, and with the phosphorylation of the LC2 light chain. Myosin belongs to a family of proteins formed by various developmentally regulated isoenzymes. This is reflected in ontogenetical changes in the ATPase activity of myosin.

The rat myocardium is formed by three isoenzymes V1-V3. Isoenzyme V3 has the lowest ATPase activity.[26] A newborn rat myocardium contains only V3. During the postnatal period there occurs the synthesis of V1 which constitutes 100% of myosin molecules at the time of weaning; the enzyme activity rises.[11,26] Between the 30th and the 60th day all three isomyosins are synthesized and the enzyme activity therefore declines (Fig. 7).

The right-to-left differences in the enzyme activity of myosin arise probably directly from different relative proportions of isomyosin V1 and V3; the concentration of V3 is lower in the right ventricle and in the right papillary muscle.[28]

The trigger for the synthesis of individual isomyosins is still a matter of discussion, the likely factors being changes in various hormones (thyroxin, catecholamines, insulin), increased circulatory demands, regulation of gene expression, etc. The composition of the myocardium determines also the velocity of contraction,[31] velocity of cross-bridge cycling and increased time of cross-bridge interaction.

A higher content of V3 reduces the velocity of shortening and economized contraction.[47] This phenomenon plays a role also in a hypoxic myocardium[30,33] and various models of the cardiac overload (for review see 23). Like the Ca-ATPase activity of myosin, the actin-activated ATPase of myosin and the K-ATPase activity of this protein change also during myocardial development.[25]

The changes are especially marked during the first postnatal weeks. Less is known about the changes in the regulatory proteins of the myofibrils:[33] troponin and tropomyosin modulate the interaction of myosin and actin in a calcium-dependent way. Tropomyosin is formed by two subunits, alpha and beta. The relative proportion of the beta component increases during the postnatal development of the myocardium and the increase is assumed to correlate with the perinatal drop in the heart rate.[34]

Troponin (Tn) consists of three subunits (TnT, TnC, TnI) which have specific biological functions.[22] Developmental changes during myocardial maturation have so far been established only in TnI.[34,35,36]

Cardiac relaxation and contraction are generally acknowledged to result from Ca uptake and release by sarcoplasmic reticulum in cardiac myocytes. The mechanism of the Ca uptake occurs through the activity of Ca- and Mg- dependent ATPase that translocates Ca from the systolic to the inner structure of the reticulum. This process could be modified via phosphorylation of phosholamban.[37]

Phosphorylation of this protein with m.w. 24 000 was first described by Krause et al.[38]

The present study shows that the Ca uptake markedly increases during myocardial development. The low value in newborns correlated well with the finding that Ca uptake as well as CaATPase activity of sarcoplasmic reticulum in fetal myocardium is low.[40,41,42] However, neither these nor other Authors[42] endeavoured to determine the time course of this parameter, comparing merely the immature myocardium with the mature one.

Biological membranes (sarcolemma, reticulum, etc) are composed of a bilayer formed by a lipid and protein component. Membrane integrity is a necessary condition for the maintenance of intracellular and extracellular ionic milieu. During the postnatal development of cardiac muscle a maturation of the membrane channel operation and ion pump system takes place.[39,41,43,44]

Marked changes occur in the phospholipid composition of the membranes.[45] We showed in our experiments[19] that the concentration of tocopherol and membrane-bound lipophilic scavengers also changes (Figs. 9,10). As tocopherol enhances membrane stability[46] it can be safely assumed that the high concentration of tocopherol, that we have found in newborn rats, along with the large pool of various hydrophobic scavengers, forms a basis of membrane integrity. Glycolytically generated ATP also plays a role.[10]

The high concentration of glycogen (Fig.11) found in newborn animals is metabolized mostly through glycolysis since mitochondria are still scarce and incompletely functional.[4]

The glycolytically generated ATP[10] contributes not only to the high resistance of newborn myocardium against acute hypoxic damage but also to the maturation and stabilization of myocardial membrane formation.

Collagenous proteins are formed by a mixture of different collagens, elastin, glycoproteins and other elements. They have an important biological role:

50

1. they form a support structure for myocytes
2. maintain a defence mechanism against invasion of foreign proteins
3. aid in nutrition of myocytes and
4. form a lubricant for contractile material.[48]

Although myocytes take up more than a half of the myocardial volume, fibroblasts represent more than 2/3 of the total cell number.[51]

The collagenous matrix is formed primarily by collagen I that aggregates into thick fibres; another component is collagen III that forms thin fibres and a minority collagen IV present in both fibroblasts and myocytes, which connects both types of cells (myocytes and fibroblasts).[50]

We have shown in this study that the relative proportion of this collagen fraction in the myocardium increases during the postnatal period. Collagen concentrations were found to be enhanced already in the early phase of the postnatal period; it can be assumed that the previously observed higher concentration of collagen in the right ventricle of adult animals results from changes occurring already in the early phase of myocardial development.[53,48,49]

As in contractile proteins, the fraction of collagenous proteins also undergoes qualitative changes. The perinatal period is characterized by a relatively high concentration of collagen III; in adulthood the relative proportion of collagen III decreases to about 20%.[48] Remodelling of existing collagen patterns is detected also during a number of different lesions of the cardiac muscle, e.g. in hypertrophic and hypoxic myocardium,[21,52,53,54] and is reflected in an increased synthesis of collagen III. Consequently, morphological remodelling of the whole collagen system in myocardium takes place not only during development, but also as a reaction to new circulatory conditions.[55]

Thick collagen fibres run parallel to muscle fibres while thin collagen fibres (coll. III) are perpendicular to thick collagen fibres.

Understanding of the changes in cardiovascular structure and function that accompany growth is a prerequisite to providing a framework within which the effects of a variety of cardiac diseases can be elucidated. Although the time course of changes taking place in a myocardium exposed to a nonphysiological damage (e.g. pressure or volume overload) will obviously differ from the time profile of ontogenetically observed changes, the sequence of the changes can be expected to be retained. Ontogenetical studies also reveal the vast plasticity and adaptive possibilities of the myocardium.

A complex view of the whole field aids not only in disclosing different biochemical mechanisms of myocardial contraction but renders it also possible to place the processes in a broader biological context.

Acknowledgement: We are grateful to Mr Vesely and Miss Mrtkova for skilled technical assistance

References

1. Bugaisky L., Zak R.: Cellular growth of cardiac muscle after birth. Tex. Rep. Biol. 1979; 39:123-138

2. Baldwin K.M., Cooke D.A., Cheadle W.G.: Enzyme alteration in neonatal heart muscle during development. J. mol. Cell. Cardiol. 1977; 9:651-660

3. Friedman W.F.: The intrinsic physiologic properties of the developing heart. Progress in Cardiovasc. Diseases 1972; 15:87-111

4. Anversa P., Ricci R., Olivetti G.: Quantitative structural analysis of the myocardium during physiologic growth and induced cardiac hypertrophy: A review. J. Am. Coll. Cardiol. 1986; 7:1140-1149

5. Mc Darmott P., Daoot M., Klein I.: Contraction regulates myosin content of cultured heart cells. Am. J. Physiol. 1985; 249:H763-H769

6. Morgan H.E., Chua B.H.L., Fuller E.O., Siehl D.: Regulation of protein synthesis and degradation during in vitro cardiac work. Am. J. Physiol. 1980; (Endocrinol. Met.) E 431-E442

7. Rakusan K.: Cardiac growth, maturation and aging. In: Zak R. (Ed.) *Growth of the heart in health and diseases.* New York, Raven 1984; 131-164

8. Engelmann G.L., Gerrity R.G.: Biochemical characterization of neonatal cardiomyocyte development in normotensive and hypertensive rats. J. Mol. Cell. Cardiol. 1988; 20:169-177

9. Massey K.D., Burton K.P.: Alpha-tocopherol attenuated myocardial membrane-related alteration resulting from ischemia and reperfusion: Am. J. Physiol. 1989; 256:H1192-H1199

10. Bricknell O.L., Opie L.H.: Effect of substrates on tissue metabolic changes in isolated rat heart during underperfusion and on release of lactate dehydrogenase and arrythmias during reperfusion. Circ. Res. 1978; 43:102-115

11. Pelouch V., Ostadal B., Prochazka J.: The ontogenetic development of ATPase activity in the right and left ventricle of the rat heart. Physiol. bohemoslov 1978; 27:268

12. Fulton R.M., Hutchinson R.M., Jones A.M.: Ventricular weight in cardiac hypertrophy. British Heart J. 1952; 14:413-420

13. World Heath Organization: Chronic cor pulmonale: Report of an expert committee: Technical Report Series N° 213. WHO Geneva 1962

14. Pelouch V., Deyl Z., Ostadal B., Wachtlova M.: Protein profiling in heart muscle. Physiol. bohemoslovaca 1984; 33:278-279

15. Lowry O.H., Rosebrough N.J., Farr A.L.: Protein measurement with Folin Phenol reagent. J. biol. Chem., 1951; 193:265-273

16. Delcayre C., Swynghedauw B.: A comparative study of heart myosin ATPase and light subunits from different species. Pflugers Arch., 1975; 255:39-47

17. Huszar G.: Monitoring of collagen and collagen fragments in chromatography of protein mixtures. Anal. Biochem. 1980; 105:424-429

18. Levitsky D.O., Aliev M.K., Kuzmin A.V., Levchenko T.S., Smirnov V.N., Chazov E.I.: Isolation of calcium pump system and purification of calcium ion dependent ATPase from heart muscle. Biochimica et Biophysica Acta, 1976; 443:468-484

19. Lebedev A.V., Sadretinov S.M., Pelouch V., Prochazka J., Levitsky D.O., Ostadal B.: Free radical membrane scavengers in myocardium of rats of different age exposed to chronic hypoxia. Biomed. Biochim. Acta 1989; 48:S122-125

20. Schrieber S.S., Rothschild M.A., Evans C., Reff F., Oratz Z.: The effect of pressure or flow stress on right ventricular protein synthesis in the face of constant and restricted coronary perfusion. J. Clin. Invest. 1975; 55:1-11

21. Jajil J.E., Doering C.W., Janicki J.S., Pick R., Shroff S.G., Weber K.: Fibrillar collagen and

myocardial stiffness in the intact hypertrophied rat left ventricle. Cir. Res. 1989; 64:1041-1050

22. Perry S.V.: The regulation of contractile activity in muscle. Bioch. Soc. Transaction 1976; 7:593-617

23. Swynghedauw B.: Developmental and functional adaptation of contractile proteins in cardiac and skeletal muscles. Physiol. Rev. 1986; 710-771

24. Medugorac I.: Alteration in myosin substructure and myofibrillar ATPase activity in rat myocardium during development and after work overload. Hoppe-Seylers Z.f. Physiol. 1979; 360:326-330

25. Watras J.: Changes in rat cardiac during development and in cure. J. mol. cell. Cardiol. 1981; 113:1011-1021

26. Hoh J.F.Y., McGrath P.A., White R.I.: Electrophoretic analysis of multiple forms of rat cardiac myosin: Effect of hypophysectomy and thyroxin. J. mol. cell. Cardiol. 1978; 10:1053-1076

27. Lompre A.M., Schwartz K., De Albis A., Lacombe G., VanThien N., Swynghedauw B.: Myosin isoenzyme redistribution in chronic heart overload. Nature 1979; 282:5-12

28. Brooks W.W., Bing O.H.L., Blaustein A.S., Allen P.D.: Comparison of contractile state and myosin isoenzymes of rat right and left ventricular myocardium. J. mol. cell. cardiol. 1987; 19:433-440

29. Bandman E.: Myosin isoenzyme transitions in muscle development, maturation, and disease. International Rev. Cytol. 1985; 97:97-131

30. Pelouch V., Ostadal B., Urbanova D., Prochazka J., Ressl J., Widimsky J.: Effect of intermittent high altitude hypoxia on the structure and enzymatic activity of cardiac myosin. Physiol. bohemoslov. 1980; 29:313-322

31. Barany M.: ATPase activity of myosin correlated with speed of muscle shortening. J. gen. Physiol. 1967; 50:197-218

32. Ostadal B., Prochazka J., Pelouch V., Urbanova D., Widimsky J.: Comparison of cardiopulmonary responses of male and female rats to intermittent high altitude hypoxia. Physiol. bohemoslov. 1984; 33:129-138

33. Humhreys J., Cummins P.: Regulatory proteins of the myocardium. Atrial and ventricular tropomyosin and troponin in the developing and adult bovine and human heart. J. mol. cell. Cardiol. 1984; 16:643-657

34. Humphreys J., Cummins P.: Regulatory proteins of the myocardium. Atrial and ventricular tropomyosin and troponin % in the developing and adult bovine and human heart. J. Mol. Cell Cardiol. 1984; 16: 643-657

35. Toyota N., Shimada Y.: Differentiation of troponin in cardiac and skeletal muscle in chicken embryos as studied by immunofluorescence microscopy. J. cell. Biol. 1981; 91:497-504

36. Dhoot G.K., Perry S.V., Vrbova G.: Changes in the distribution of components of the troponin complex. Exp. Neurol. 1981; 72:513-530

37. Tada M., Katz A.M.: Phoshorylation of the sarcoplasmic reticulum and sarcolemma. Annu. Rev. Physiol. 1982; 44:401-433

38. Krause E-G., Will H., Pelouch V., Wollenberger A.: Cyclic AMP-dependent protein kinase activity in a cell membrane enriched subcellular fraction of pig myocardium. Acta Biol. Med. Germ. 1973; 31:k37-43

39. Levitsky D.O., Syrbu S.I., Cherepakhin V., Rokhlin O.V.: Mononuclear antibodies to dog heart sarcoplasmic reticulum. Europ. J. Biochem. 1987

40. Naraysanan N.: Comparison of ATP-dependent calcium transport and calcium activated ATPase activities of cardiac sarcoplasmic reticulum and sarcolemma from rats of various ages. Mechanisms of Ageing and development 1987; 38:127-143

41. Pegg W., Michalak M.: Differentiation of sarcoplasmic reticulum during cardiac myogenesis.

Am. J. Physiol. 252 (Heart Circ. Physiol.) 1987; H22-H31

42. Michalak M.: Identification of Ca-release activity and ryanodine receptor in sarcoplasmic-reticulum membranes during cardiac myogenesis. Biochem. J. 1988; 253:631-636

43. Will H., Kuttner I., Vetter R., Will-Shahab L., Kemsies Ch.: Early presence of phosholamban in developing chick heart. FEBS letters. 1983; 155:326-330

44. Chamberlain B.K., Levitsky D.O., Fleischner S.: Isolation and characterization of canine cardiac sarcoplasmic reticulum with improved Ca-transport properties. J. Biol. Chem. 1983; 258:6602-6609

45. Chien K.B., Han A., Sen L., Buja L.M., Willerson J.T.: Accumulation of unesterified arachidonic acid in ischemic canine myocardium: relationship to a phosphatidylcholine deacylation cycle and the depletion of membrane phospholipids. Circ. Res. 1984; 54:313-322

46. Lucy J.A.: Functional and structural aspects of biological membranes: a suggested structural role of vitamin E in control of membrane permeability and stability. Ann. NY Acad. Sci. 1972; 203:4-11

47. Alpert N.R., Mullieri L.A.: Increased myothermal economy of isometric force generation in compensated cardiac hypertrophy induced by pulmonary artery constriction in the rabbit. Circ. Res. 1982; 50:491-500

48. Weber K.. Cardiac interstitium in health and disease: The fibrillar collagen network. J. Am. Coll. Cardiol. 1989; 13:1637-1652

49. Ostadal B., Mirejovska E., Hurych J., Pelouch V., Prochazka J.: Effect of intermittent high altitude hypoxia on the synthesis of collagenous and non-collagenous proteins of the right and left ventricular myocardium. Cardiovascular Res. 1978; 12:303-308

50. Eghbali M., Czaja M.J., Zedel M., Weiner F.R., Zern M.A., Seifter S., Blumenfeld O.O.: Collagen chain mRNAs in isolated heart cells from young and adult rats. J. mol. cell. cardiol. 1988; 20:267-276

51. Zak R.: Development and proliferative capacity of cardiac muscle cells. Circ. Revs. Suppl. II. 1974; 17-26

52. Pelouch V., Ostadal B., Prochazka J.: The effect of hypoxia on the structural and enzymatic properties of cardiac myosin. Abhandlungen der Akad. Wissenschaften DDR, 1987; 215-218

53. Pelouch V., Ostadal B., Prochazka J., Urbanova D., Widimsky J.: Effect of high altitude hypoxia on the protein composition of the right ventricular myocardium in young rats. In: Daum S. (Ed.) *Interaction between heart and lung* . Stuttgart-New York, Georg Thieme Verlag 1989; 69-72

54. Medugorac I., Jacob R.: Characterization of left ventricular collagen in the rat. Cardiovasc. Res. 1983; 17:15-21

55. Speir E., Yi-Fu Z., Lee M., Shrivastav S., Casscells W.: Fibroblast growth factors are presented in adult cardiac myocytes, in vivo. Biochem. Biophys. Res. Comm. 1988; 157:1136-1340

5. Hypoxia-Induced Right Ventricular Aneurysm

L.C. Ou[1], N.S. Hill[2], B.P. Pickett[1], C.S. Faulkner[1], G.L. Sardella[1], C.D. Thron[1], S.M. Tenney[1]

1. *Departments of Physiology, Pathology, Pharmacology and Toxicology, Dartmouth Medical School, Hanover, NH, USA*
2. *Pulmonary Division, Rhode Island Hospital, Providence, RI, USA*

Supported by a grant (HL-21159) from the National Heart, Lung and Blood Institute

Introduction

Aneurysm is a permanent abnormal dilatation of an artery or ventricle resulting from localized structural weakness and stretching of the arterial or ventricular wall due to high transmural pressure. Aneurysms occur mainly in systemic arteries and, to a lesser extent, in the left ventricle.

Aneurysms of the main pulmonary artery or its branches are rare and right ventricular aneurysms (RVA) have not been reported. Recently, we found that RVA develops in Madison (M) but not in Hilltop (H) rats following chronic exposure to hypoxia.[1]

Since RVA does not occur in either strain of rats under normoxic control conditions, it seemed likely that the hypoxic exposure was involved in the pathogenesis of RVA.

Since the right ventricle is a thin-walled structure suitable for pumping blood through the low pressure, low resistance pulmonary circuit and is vulnerable to pressure overloading,[2] the RVA could be the result of the hypoxia-induced pulmonary arterial hypertension. Although this could occur in either strain of rats, M and H rats differ substantially in their vasoresponsiveness to hypoxia;[3] early during hypoxia (24-48 h), pulmonary arterial pressure (Ppa) rises abruptly and considerably more in M rats.

Since RVA is observed only in M rats, it is possible that this initial abrupt severe rise in Ppa is critical in the pathogenesis of hypoxia-induced RVA (HRVA). If so, it is also possible that any agent or treatment which suppresses the rise in Ppa during acute hypoxia would prevent HRVA.

The aims of the present study were:
1. to describe the pathological process of HRVA formation,
2. to test the proposed cause and prevention of HRVA, and
3. to examine the influence of sex on the pathogenesis of HRVA.

Materials and Methods

Sprague-Dawley male and female rats, weighing 220-300 g, were obtained from Hilltop, Scottdale, PA (H) and Madison, WI (M) breeding laboratories. Both hypobaric (simulated high altitude) and normobaric (low oxygen content at sea level pressure) hypoxia were employed in the present study. No distinction in the results could be made between these two modes of hypoxia. A hypobaric chamber was used for hypoxic exposures longer than 1 h and normobaric hypoxia was used for shorter exposures. The two strains of rat were placed in the same hypoxic chamber at 24-26°C or were maintained under normoxic conditions in the same laboratory.[3,4]

Exposure of animals to 10.5% O_2 for 30 days was the basic experimental procedure used to induce HRVA. Since the severe acute rise in Ppa that occurs in hypoxic M rats lasts only for the initial 24-48 h of hypoxia,[3] experimental manipulations used to alter this initial pressure rise were introduced during the early period (first 3 days) of hypoxia.

A. Major series of experiments

Series 1 was designed to determine the pulmonary pressor response to acute hypoxia in fully awake H and M rats. Three levels of hypoxia (14,10.5 and 8.5% O_2) were tested.

One or two days prior to measurements, each rat was prepared with an indwelling pulmonary arterial catheter according to the procedure described previously.[3] During measurements, each rat was placed in a clear plastic restraining cage through which ambient room air or hypoxic gases could be flushed. The pulmonary arterial catheter was connected to a Statham pressure transducer (P23) and Ppa was continuously monitored on a Grass Model 7 polygraph. During a 10 min period, the rat was exposed to a low oxygen gas mixture and the rise in Ppa from the mean baseline value (recorded at 20.9% O_2) was recorded.

Series 2 was designed to evaluate the effects of exposing rats to different oxygen levels during the early period of chronic hypoxia. Control groups of both H and M rats were exposed to 10.5% O_2 for 30 days.

Experimental rats were first exposed for 3 days at either 14 or 8.5% O_2 and then exposed for 27 days at 10.5% O_2. At the end of the chronic exposure period, right ventricular peak systolic pressure (RVPP) was measured in both the control and experimental groups under anaesthesia.[4,5] The rats were then sacrificed and examined for the presence of RVA. The severity of pathology was estimated from the size (area) of each RVA.

Series 3 was designed to evaluate the effects of administering a vasodilator (nifedipine or verapamil) during the early period of chronic hypoxia. Two control groups were studied; one received DMSO and the other received saline. One experimental group received nifedipine (10 mg/kg in dimethyl sulphoxide (DMSO), i.p.) and another received verapamil (10 mg/kg in saline i.p.). In all animals, exposure to hypoxia was begun immediately after the first injection of drug. Injections were repeated every 4 h for a total of 6 injections (24 h) and the hypoxia was continued for 30 days. Each animal was then assessed for HRVA.

Series 4 was designed to determine the effects of exposure to short duration hypoxia without chronic hypoxia. One group of 6 male M rats was exposed to 10.5% O_2 for 3 days and then to normoxia for 27 days.

B. Additional series of experiments

Series 5 was designed to examine structural characteristics of the right ventricles from H and M rats exposed to normoxic (control) and hypoxic conditions. After sacrificing the rats, the hearts were placed in 10% formalin. The ventricles were then cut longitudinally into 4 μn thick sections, embedded in paraffin, and stained with haematoxylin and eosin.

These sections were examined using light microscopy.

Following the observation that M rats initially exposed to mild hypoxia (14% O_2) for 3 days did not develop HRVA, two additional series of experiments were designed. In the first, M rats were exposed to 3 days of mild hypoxia (14% O_2). These rats were then sacrificed and the ventricles were weighed in order to detect the presence of hypertrophy. In the second, Ppa responses to acute brief (10-20 min) exposures to severe hypoxia (10.5% O_2) were measured in rats being exposed to mild hypoxia (14% O_2) for 3 days. This series was done to determine whether the latter suppressed the acute pressure responses.

Series 6 was designed to explore the influence of sex. The incidence and severity of HRVA in male and female H and M rats exposed to severe or mild hypoxia were examined. In addition, the relationship between pulmonary pressor responses and different levels of acute hypoxia was studied in male and female M rats.

Statistical analysis

Statistical methods followed Snedecor[6] or Siegel.[7] Differences are reported as statistically significant when the p values were < 0.05.

58

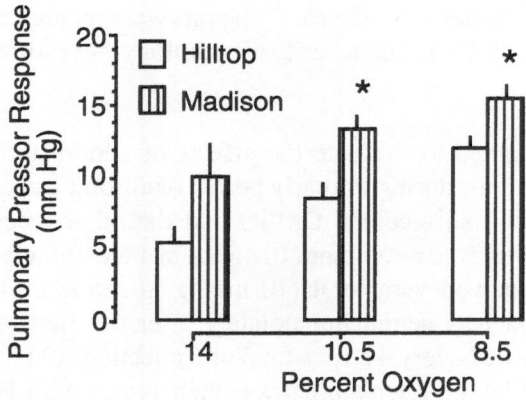

Fig. 1. Dose-response relationships of pulmonary pressor responses to acute hypoxia in male M and H rats. Data are means ± SEM from 5 animals of each strain. Asterisks denote P-value <0.05 for comparison between the two strains at that level of hypoxia.

Results

Effects of acute hypoxia on pulmonary arterial pressure

Hypoxic pulmonary pressor responses increased as the intensity of the acute hypoxic stimulus was increased in male H and M rats. The responses were greater in M than in H rats for each level of hypoxia (Fig. 1). These observations confirm and extend the findings from previous studies reported from this laboratory.[3]

Effects of exposure to different oxygen levels during the early period of chronic hypoxia

As shown in Table I, HRVA was found in 50% of the M rats and in none of the H rats exposed to 10.5% O_2 for 30 days. When exposed to more severe hypoxia (8.5% O_2) for 3 days and then exposed to 10.5% O_2 for 27 days, the incidence of HRVA in M rats was increased to 75%. A small but well-defined HRVA was seen in one H rat. In contrast, no HRVA was observed in the rats initially exposed to 14% O_2 for 3 days before being exposed to 10.5% O_2 for 27 days.

These findings in conjunction with those shown in figure 1 indicate that incidence of HRVA was directly related to the severity of the acute pulmonary pressor responses associated with the early period of hypoxia. In contrast, the incidence of HRVA was unrelated to the severity of the chronic pulmonary hypertension associated with the late period of hypoxia. In particular, the final steady-state RVPP in the group of rats initially exposed to mild hypoxia (14% O_2) was considerably greater than in the rats from the other two groups exposed initially to severe hypoxia (one group at 10.5% O_2 for 30 days, the other at 8.5% O_2 for 3

Table I. Effects of initial exposures (3 days) to mild (14% O_2) and severe (8.5% O_2) hypoxia on the incidence and severity of HRVA.[a]

Groups	Incidence (%)	Severity (mm²)	RVPP (mmHg)
M-14 (7)	0/7 (0)	0	84.1±1.2
M-10.5 (8)	4/8 (50)[b]	68.7±30.9	58.8±4.3[c]
M-8.5 (7)	5/7 (70)[b]	68.4±11.9	58.9±4.0[c]
H-10.5 (10)	0/10 (0)	0	93.1±3.0
H-8.5 (10)	1/10 (10)	~1-2	94.2±3.9

[a] Control groups (M-10.5 and H-10.5) were exposed to hypoxia (10.5% O_2) for 30 days. M-14, M-8.5, and H-8.5 groups were exposed to 14 and 8.5% O_2, respectively, for the first 3 days and then to 10.5% O_2 for 27 days. Figures in parentheses are number of animals studied. Severity of HRVA is expressed as the total surface area in mm². RVPP = right ventricular peak systolic pressure.
[b] The incidence of HRVA in M rats was significantly higher in the M-10.5 and M-8.5 groups than in the M-14 group (p<0.05, Fisher test).
[c] The RVPP was significantly lower in the M-8.5 and M-10.5 groups than in the M-14 groups (t-test).

days and then at 10.5% O_2 for 27 days). It was the latter two groups with the lower RVPP values that developed RVA. Moreover, RVPP was much greater in H rats than in M rats, yet only one of the H rats developed RVA and this occurred at the most severe level of hypoxia.

The early exposure to mild hypoxia (14% O_2 for 3 days) resulted in an increase in the ratio of right ventricular weight to body weight from a control value of 0.051±0.001 to a value of 0.058±0.001 (SEM, N = 6; p<0.01, t-test). Also, the ratio of right ventricular weight to left ventricular plus septal weights increased from a control value of 0.25±0.01 to a value of 0.28±0.01 (SEM, N = 6; p<0.01, t-test). The early mild hypoxic exposure enhanced, rather than suppressed, the acute pulmonary pressor responses produced at the onset of subsequent exposure to severe hypoxia (10.5% O_2).

Figure 2 shows the development of this enhanced responsiveness during the 3-day mild hypoxic exposure. Despite this enhanced pressor responsiveness to hypoxia, these animals did not develop RVA (Tables I and III).

Effects of administering vasodilators during the early period of chronic hypoxia

In agreement with previous studies,[8] nifedipine or verapamil, at a dose of 10 mg/kg, i.p., inhibited acute hypoxic pulmonary pressor responses in conscious rats. Control responses without nifedipine were 13.5±0.6 mmHg, responses with nifedipine were 2.5±0.2 mmHg (SEM, N = 4, p<0.01, t-test); control responses without verapamil were 14.0±0.7 mmHg, responses with verapamil were 2.4±0.1 mmHg (SEM, N = 4, p<0.01, t-test).

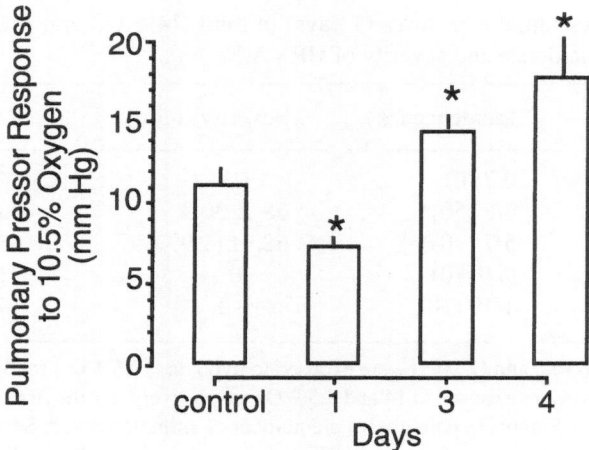

Fig. 2. Effects of exposure to mild hypoxia on pulmonary pressor responses to severe hypoxia in male M rats. Rats were exposed to 14% O_2 and their pulmonary pressor responses to 10.5% O_2 were tested after different time intervals at mild hypoxia. Data are means ± SEM from 4 animals. Asterisks denote P-value <0.05 for comparison with the control values (t test). Control values (C) were measured prior to exposure to mild hypoxia.

Table II. Effects of 24h treatments with nifedipine or verapamil on incidence of HRVA after 30 days of hypoxia.

Groups	Incidence (%)	Mortality
M-C (6)	3/4 (75)	2*
M-Ve (6)	0/5 (0)	1*
M-Ni (6)	0/6 (0)	0

All groups of animals were exposed to 10.5% O_2 for 30 days. M-C is the control group, half of which were given saline and the other half DMSO. M-Ve and M-Ni are experimental groups, treated with verapamil and nifedipine respectively every 4h for the first 24h of hypoxia. Figures in parentheses are number of animals studied. The incidence of HRVA in survivors was significantly higher in the control groups than in either drug-treated group (p<0.05, Fisher test).
* Deaths occurred in the first two days of hypoxic exposure.

Administration of solvents for either nifedipine (DMSO) or verapamil (saline) produced no changes in pressor responsiveness. The duration of inhibition produced by both agents was > 4 h (6-24 h). Thus, injecting every 4 h was considered sufficient in order to suppress pulmonary vascular responsiveness throughout the 24 h administration period.

None of the M rats in which either nifedipine or verapamil was administered

Table III. Incidence and severity of HRVA in males and females of both M and H strains of rats after 30 days of hypoxia

Groups	Incidence	Severity (mm)	RVPP (mmHg)
M_m-10.5 (6)	6/6 (100)	26.01±13.3	45.3±1.5
M_f- 10.5 (6)	3/6 (50)	6.9 ± 2.5	45.7±3.8
H_m-10.5 (6)	0/6 (0)	-	80.0±4.1
H_f- 10.5 (6)	0/6 (0)	-	75.6±3.5
M_m-14 (6)	0/6 (0)	-	56.0±1.9
M_f- 14 (6)	0/6 (0)	-	51.8±2.1

All groups were exposed to 10.5% O_2 for 30 days except M_m-14 and M_f-14 groups that were exposed to 14% O_2 for the first 3 days and to 10.5% O_2 for the remaining 27 days. M_m, M_f, H_m, H_f are males and females of M and H rats. Figures in parentheses in first column are number of animals studied. RVPP = right ventricular peak systolic pressure. Severity of HRVA is expressed as the total surface area in mm^2. For the M_m-10.5 and M_f-10.5 groups, a statistically significant difference in the severity of HRVA was found by the median test, with the 3 females without HRVA counted as severity < 1 mm.

developed HRVA (Table II). Two animals from a control group and one from the verapamil-treated group died during the first 2 days of hypoxia. Acute right ventricular failure due to a severe rise in Ppa in response to acute hypoxia was thought not to be responsible for the death in the verapamil-treated group since this agent probably suppressed the hypoxic pulmonary pressor response.

Effects of exposure to brief severe hypoxia without chronic exposure to hypoxia
    HRVA was found in 50% (3/6) of the M rats exposed for 3 days at 10.5% O_2 and then 27 days at normoxia. The size of these lesions was smaller than those seen in the male M rats exposed to 10.5% O_2 for 30 days (Tables I and III). With respect to the incidence of HRVA, these results are not statistically different than those from the group of M rats exposed to 10.5% O_2 for 30 days. Preliminary observations showed that 3 days of severe hypoxia (10.5% O_2) was sufficient to produce myocytolysis.

Influence of sex
    As shown in Table III, exposure to 10.5% O_2 for 30 days induced HRVA in all male but in only 50% of the female M rats. Because of the small numbers, this difference is not statistically significant. HRVA was more severe in males than in females. Under the same hypoxic conditions, no HRVA developed in male or female H rats.
    Following chronic hypoxia (30 days at 10.5% O_2), mean RVPP was markedly

elevated but was significantly lower in the M than H rats with no sex differences discernible. These findings corroborate our previous studies[5] and provide supporting evidence that the magnitude of RVPP during chronic hypoxia was not the determining factor in the development of HRVA. We also exposed female and male M rats to 14% O_2 for 3 days and then to 10.5% O_2 for 27 days.

Consistent with the preceding studies, this early exposure to mild hypoxia prevented HRVA from occurring in either sex. As seen in Table III, the incidence of HRVA dropped to zero.

Acute pulmonary pressor responses increased with increasing severity of hypoxia in both male and female M rats. There were no sex differences at each level of hypoxia tested. The duration of these hypoxic pressor responses in the two sexes was not examined.

Histological changes associated with HRVA

A moderately severe HRVA is shown in figure 3. The lesions occurred primarily in the upper region of the right ventricle; small ones appeared near the pulmonary outflow tract and large ones extended into the lateral wall and septum. Sizes of HRVA varied from barely detectable to as large as two thirds of the whole ventricle and protruded in situ like a balloon during a systole. Histologically, the afflicted

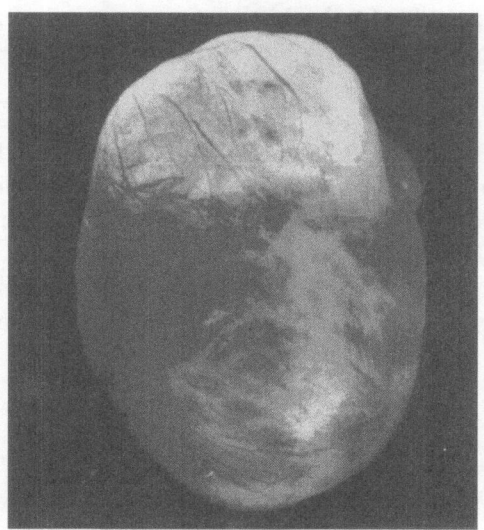

Fig. 3. A pathograph of a heart freshly obtained from a male M rat following 30 days exposure to hypoxia (10.5% O_2). The right ventricle was inflated with saline. Note the marked HRVA. The bright spot at the bottom was artifact due to polyethylene tubing used for inflation with saline.

right ventricular free wall showed evidence of injury ranging from subendocardial foci of myocytolysis to extensive transmural replacement fibrosis with thinning of the wall and frank aneurysm formation.

The histological appearance of the ventricles did not differ between control H and M rats. Following exposure to hypoxia for varying durations, right ventricular hypertrophy was always greater in H than that in M rats. Pathologically, both left and right ventricles showed signs of ischaemia including the presence of atrophic and necrotic myocytes, patches of increased interstitial cellularity, foci of extravasated red blood cells and increased density of Anitschkow cells. These changes increased with the duration of hypoxia and were appreciably more extensive in H than in M rats. However, even in the H rats, these ischaemic lesions were relatively mild and undoubtedly did not produce significant haemodynamic effects.[9]

Discussion

The present study demonstrates the development of HRVA in rats exposed to severe chronic hypoxia. Grossly, these aneurysms consist of thin-walled outpouchings that originate near the pulmonary outflow tract and vary in extent from barely recognizable to two-thirds of the right ventricular free wall. Histologically, they consist of a fibrous membrane that replaces the normal myocardium.

Because the HRVA occurs almost exclusively in M rats which at the onset of chronic hypoxia show a vigorous though transient pulmonary pressor response,[3] we postulated that the magnitude of this acute pressor response could be important in triggering early pathological changes within the right ventricle and that these changes could later lead to the development of HRVA. Evidence presented in this report supports this hypothesis. First, when the initial pressor response is enhanced by an extreme hypoxic stimulus (8.5% O_2), the incidence of HRVA increases. Second, when the initial pressor response is diminished by a mild hypoxic stimulus (14% O_2), the incidence of HRVA is reduced to zero. Third, when the initial pressor response is inhibited by vasodilator agents (e.g., nifedipine and verapamil), the incidence of HRVA is reduced to zero. Fourth, and perhaps most remarkable, small but well-defined HRVA occur when M rats are exposed to only 3 days of severe hypoxia (10.5% O_2) without subsequent chronic hypoxia. This finding clearly points to the importance of the pathological changes produced during the early period of hypoxia.

Myocardial hypertrophy develops in M rats exposed to only 3 days of mild hypoxia (14% O_2). If these animals are then subjected to chronic severe hypoxia (27 days at 10.5% O_2), they do not develop HRVA even though the acute pulmonary pressor responsiveness to severe hypoxia is greatly enhanced (Fig. 2). It would appear that early development of hypertrophy prevents or protects against pathological changes that lead to HRVA. Perhaps during the early period of hypoxia,

64

there is a critical balance between constructive cellular changes which lead to hypertrophy and destructive cellular changes which set the stage for subsequent dilatation and aneurysm formation. During mild hypoxia, the balance may favour hypertrophy; during severe hypoxia, the balance may favour dilatation. Clearly, the crucial determinant of this balance could well be the degree of the pressure load imposed on the right heart during the initial period of hypoxia.

Under the best of conditions, the right ventricle is a highly compliant, low pressure pump which tolerates increased pressure loads poorly.[2] A severe increase in right ventricular pressure has been shown to compromise right ventricular coronary blood flow, causing tissue ischaemia and eventually right ventricular failure.[10] Severe reduction in coronary blood flow due to a marked hypoxic pulmonary pressor response may cause similar ischaemia and account for subsequent HRVA formation. Delineation of the precise mechanisms which are triggered during early hypoxia and eventually lead to HRVA requires further study. Undoubtedly, these mechanisms are related to myocardial ischaemia and, since acute severe increases in Ppa occur in a variety of clinical states (e.g., acute hypoxic lung disease, acute high altitude exposure, and acute pulmonary embolism), delineation of these mechanisms will surely have important clinical implications.

References

1. Ou L.C., Sardella G.L., Hill N.S., Tenney S.M.: Right ventricular aneurysm induced by hypoxia. Proc. International Union of Physiol. Sci. 1986; 16:341
2. Abel F.L., Waldhausen J.A.: Effects of alterations in pulmonary vascular resistance on right ventricular function. J. Thoracic and Cardiovascular Surg. 1967; 54:886-894
3. Ou L.C., Sardella G.L., Hill N.S., Tenney S.M.: Acute and chronic pulmonary pressor responses to hypoxia: the role of blunting in acclimatization. Respir. Physiol. 1986; 64:81-91
4. Ou L.C., Smith R.P.: Probable strain differences of rats in susceptibilities and cardiopulmonary responses to chronic hypoxia. Respir. Physiol. 1983; 53:367-377
5. Ou L.C., Smith R.P.: Strain and sex differences in the cardiopulmonary adaption of rats to high altitude. Proc. Soc. Exp. Biol. Med. 1984; 177:308-311
6. Snedecor G.W., Cochran W.G.: *Statistical methods*. The Iowa State University Press, 7th edition 1980
7. Siegel S.: Nonparametric statistics for the behavioral sciences, New York, McGraw-Hill book Company, 1956
8. Stanbrook H.S., Morris K.G., McMurtry I.F.: Prevention and reversal of hypoxic pulmonary hypertension by calcium antagonists. Am. Rev. Resp. Dis. 1984; 130:81-85
9. Pickett B.P., Faulkner C.S., Ou L.C.: Gross and light microscopic study of myocardium in rats susceptible and resistant to chronic mountain sickness (CMS). Fourth Banff International Symposium on Hypoxia. Alberta, Canada 1985
10. Vlahakes G.J., Turley K., Hoffman J.I.E.: The pathophysiology of failure in acute right ventricular hypertension: Hemodynamic and biochemical correlations. Circulation 1981; 63:87-95

6. Study of the Factors Concurring in the Determination of Right Ventricular Hypertrophy in Chronic Obstructive Lung Disease

L. BERTOLI[1], A. MANTERO[2], C. ALLI[1], M. TAMPONI[3], R. ALPAGO[2], A. MOLINO[1], A. PEZZANO[2]

1. Vergani Medical Division, Niguarda Cà Granda Hospital, Milan, Italy
2. Cardiology Department, Niguarda Cà Granda Hospital, Milan, Italy
3. Physical Therapy Department, Niguarda Cà Granda Hospital, Milan, Italy

Introduction

As already recognized, the most important pathogenetic mechanisms inducing abnormalities in the right ventricular structure are pulmonary hypertension and abnormal concentrations of blood gases.[1] Any theory concerning the development of cor pulmonale should take account of the effects of the anatomical loss of pulmonary vessels, pulmonary arterial constrictions secondary to alveolar hypoxia and acidosis as well as of the effects of increased blood viscosity and increased blood flow.[2] However, their relative roles and the pathogenetic sequences inducing right ventricular hypertrophy (RVH) are unknown.

Though pulmonary arterial hypertension and RVH are closely related, their linking elements are poorly understood; indeed, it is necessary to understand more about the relationship existing between the extent and duration of pulmonary hypertension and the development of detectable RVH.[3,4]

Thus, the aim of our present study was to detect the main variables which may justify their role in the development of RVH in patients affected with chronic obstructive lung disease (COLD).

Materials and Methods

The present study was performed on 73 patients - only 3 were women - who suffered from COLD as defined by the WHO[5], and were aged between 37 and 74 years (mean age 56.5±8.3 years).

Table I. The 23 variables (mean values ± SD) in the patients with (group I) and without (group II) right ventricular hypertrophy (Student's t test for unpaired data)

	Group I RVAWT > 5mm	Group II RVAWT ≤ 5mm	P Value
pH	7.39±0.03	7.40±0.02	< 0.05
PaO_2 (mmHg)	58.40±11.80	66.00±11.50	< 0.001
$PaCO_2$ (mmHg)	48.30±10.10	46.50±10.10	NS
$P\bar{v}O_2$ (mmHg)	36.00±5.50	41.40±8.60	< 0.01
SaO_2 (%)	86.90±7.90	91.60±5.10	< 0.01
Hb (g/100 ml)	16.30±2.10	16.08±2.05	NS
Ht (%)	52.60±8.20	49.50±5.30	NS
H (cm)	166.90±6.10	163.10±6.90	NS
Weight (Kg)	70.60±14.40	63.50±14.80	NS
Age (yr)	55.80±8.30	58.10±8.90	NS
BMI (kgx1.000/cm)	2.50±0.50	2.30±0.40	NS
BS (m²)	1.76±0.20	1.67±0.20	NS
FEV_1 (%)	32.20±15.70	44.40±25.60	NS
$\dot{V}O_2$ (ml/min)	303.70±87.80	262.90±38.60	NS
IVS (mm)	9.80±2.80	7.60±1.20	< 0.05
RVI (mm/m²)	21.80±5.90	16.30±2.40	< 0.001
PAP (mmHg)	25.80±10.10	22.60±5.50	< 0.05
PAPs (mmHg)	43.30±18.80	59.70±26.50	NS
RVPSP (mmHg)	39.90±14.70	35.20±6.50	< 0.05
RVEDP (mmHg)	7.30±3.70	7.00±3.20	NS
WP (mmHg)	8.20±2.20	8.90±2.20	NS
CI (1/min/m²)	3.90±1.30	4.10±1.60	NS
TPR (dyn/s/cm⁻⁵)	347.20±19.80	311.70±123.40	NS

RVAWT = right ventricular arterior wall thickness;
pH = arterial pH; PaO_2 = arterial oxygen tension;
$PaCO_2$ = arterial carbon dioxide tension;
$P\bar{v}O_2$ = mixed venous oxygen tension;
SaO_2 = arterial oxygen saturation;
Hb = haemoglobin; Ht = haematocrit;
H = height; BMI = body mass index;
BS = body surface;
$\dot{V}O_2$ = oxygen consumption;
FEV_1 = forced expiratory volume in 1 sec;
IVS = interventricular septum;
RVI = diameter of the right ventricular cavity corrected by body surface;
PAP = pulmonary artery mean pressure;
PAPs = pulmonary artery systolic pressure;
RVPSP = right ventricular peak systolic pressure;
RVEDP = right ventricular end diastolic pressure;
WP = mean wedge pressure;
 CI = cardiac index; TPR = total pulmonary resistance.

These patients were all in a steady state of the disease defined by stable body weight, stable FEV_1 and arterial blood gas tensions, absence of acute respiratory infection or peripheral oedema for 3 weeks prior to the study.

All the patients showed hypoxaemia with a notable degree of airway obstruction. Most of them had pulmonary hypertension (PAP > 20 mmHg) with normal wedge capillary pressure and normal cardiac index (Table I).

Patients with other pulmonary diseases, systemic arterial hypertension (systolic pressure $\geq$ 160 mmHg and diastolic pressure $\geq$ 95 mmHg) or valvular heart or coronary artery disease were excluded from the study.

Right heart haemodynamics were performed at rest on supine patients with 5 or 7 French Swan-Ganz flow-directed catheters. Pressure values were measured with a Statham P23D transducer and recorded on a Thomson Telco recorder. The readings were taken 20-30 mins after the placing of the catheter in the pulmonary artery. Other technical indications are given elsewhere.[6]

Prior informed consent had been obtained from all the patients.

The day after the haemodynamic test, the patients were submitted to 2D-echocardiography using Ekoline '5500 D' (3.5 MHz transducer).

All the studies began with the patients in the supine position. Whenever it was impossible to obtain good images in this position, the patient was placed in a left lateral decubitus. Images were visualized in the position which allowed the best definition of the anatomical structure to be studied.

Following Weyman's indications[7], we attempted to visualize the right heart through the following approaches (views from which the various diameters were measured):

- *apical approach*: "four chamber" view;
- *parasternal approach*: "long axis of the right ventricular outflow tract" view; "short axis at the tricuspid valve level" view;
- *subcostal approach*: "long axis of the heart" view; "long axis of the right ventricular outflow tract (RVOT)" view.

By the latter approach, we selected the single optimal beam from among the many available ones. This beam was positioned exactly above the papillary muscle on a level with the tricuspid valve tendon chords (Fig. 1). We then transformed the 2D-echo into M mode, thus measuring the thickness of the right ventricular anterior wall (RVAWT) and of the interventricular septum (IVS) (Fig. 2). All the measurements were performed at end diastole defined as the frame closest to the onset of the R-wave of the electrocardiogram. The right ventricular cavity dimension, the right ventricular wall and the interventricular septum thickness were measured from the leading edge to the leading edge of the endocardial or epicardial signals. Three values for each dimension or thickness were taken from three consecutive

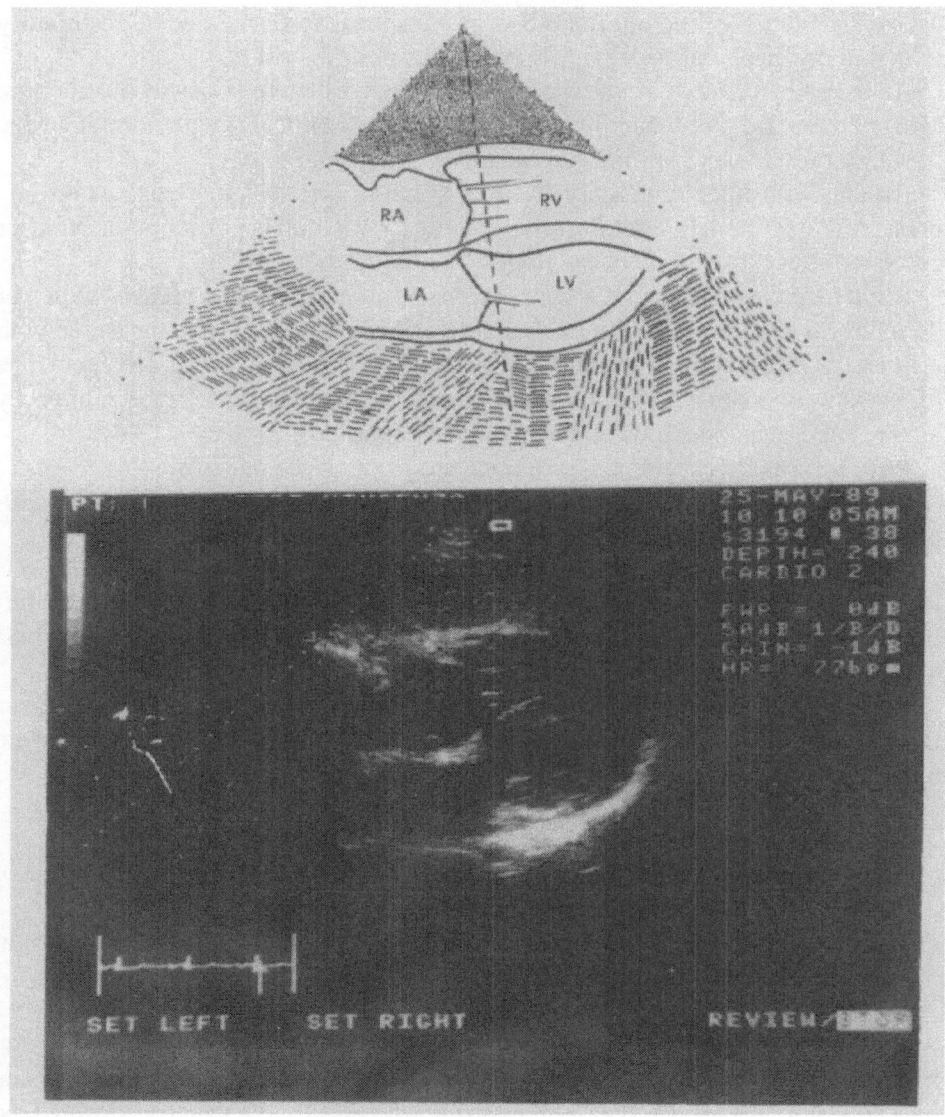

Fig. 1. Subcostal approach: long axis of the heart.
RA = right atrium;
RV = right ventricle;
LA = left atrium;
LV = left ventricle

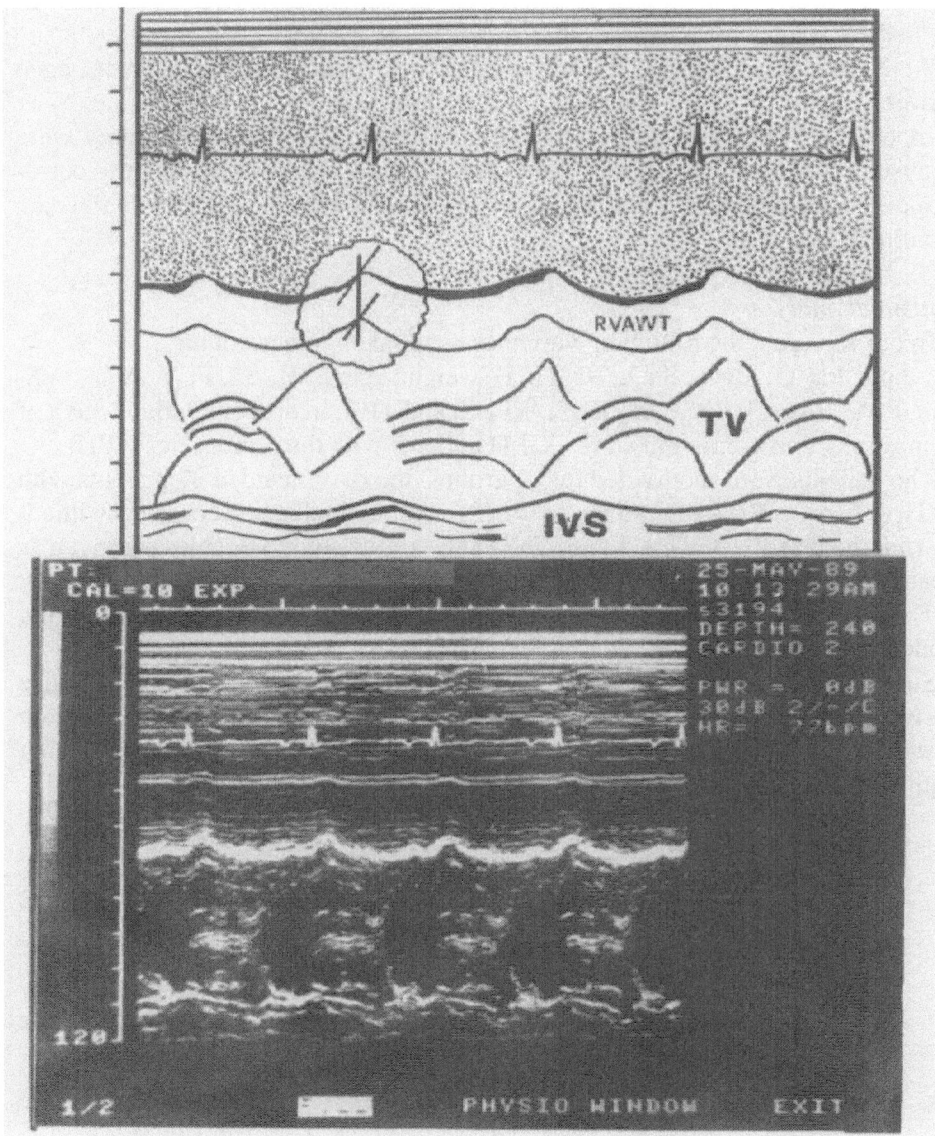

Fig. 2. M-mode subcostal approach.
RVAWT = right ventricular anterior wall thickness;
TV = tricuspid valve;
IVS = interventricular septum.

70

cardiac cycles. The measurements were averaged and the resulting datum was applied for statistical analysis.

At the same time, a 2D-echo study was performed on 24 normal subjects, aged between 37 and 58 years, considered as the control group.

In order to assess interobserver variability, the 2D-echocardiograms were analysed by two of the Authors, independently and without knowing the corresponding haemodynamic data. The probability level was $P < 0.04$ for all the data examined.

Statistical analyses

In our research, the following variables were taken into account:
pH, PaO_2. $PaCO_2$, $P\bar{v}O_2$, SaO_2, Hb, Ht, H, weight, age, BMI, BS, FEV_1, $\dot{V}O_2$, IVS, RVI, $\overline{PAP}$, PAPs, RVPSP, RVEDP, $\overline{WP}$, CI and TPR, in order to define which of them were significantly linked in COLD patients with the presence of RVH.

The patients were subdivided into 2 groups: the first included 37 patients with RVH, defined as RVAWT > 5 mm; the second group included 22 patients without RVH defined as RVAWT ≤ 5 mm. The values of the study variables are given as mean ± S.D.

The significance of the differences between mean values was tested applying Student's t test for unpaired data.

Subsequently, multiple regression analysis was carried out with the stepwise (forward and backward) selection method in order to detect the most significant parameter explaining the variability of RVAWT by optimizing the 3 following requisites:

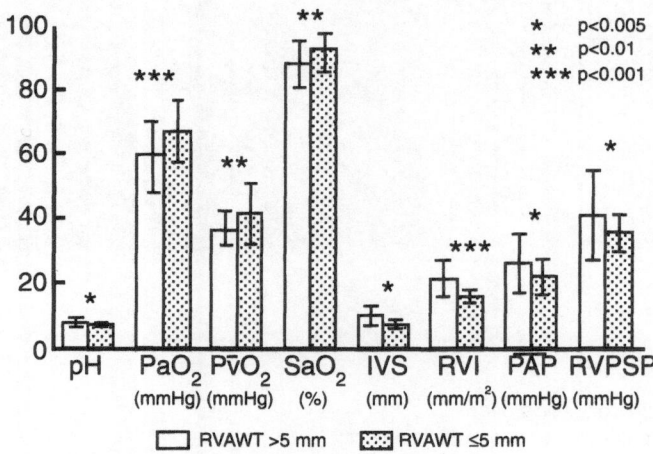

Fig. 3. Variables which turned out to be significant in distinguishing the patients with or without RVH.

a. minimization of the estimated standard error,

b. maximization of the adjusted correlation coefficient,

c. minimization of the number of necessary variables.

Going on with the statistical calculation, we used as starting variables those which turned out to be significant at the Student's t test for unpaired data, with threshold < 5% (Fig. 3). Continuing with the stepwise selection (backward and forward), we put in the above variables but the echocardiographic data IVS and RVI. For such analyses we used the statistical package Software Stat graphics.

Results

Through the subcostal approach, the RVAW was visualized to such an extent that reliable measurements could be achieved in 81% of the cases. In COLD patients, RVAWT values achieved 6.0 ± 1.9 mm, that is they were significantly higher (p<0.001) than in control patients for whom RVAWT values attained 4.0 ± 1.5 mm.

Table I shows the averages of the anthropometric, blood gas analysis, respiratory function, haemodynamic and echocardiographic variables examined in the two groups of patients. From the analysis, it appeared that the blood gas anlysis variables PaO_2, $P\overline{v}O_2$, and SaO_2 as well as pH, the echocardiographic variables IVS and RVI, and the haemodynamic variables $\overline{PAP}$ and RVPSP significantly differ in the two groups (Fig. 3). In particular, in comparison with the patients not affected from RVH, the patients with such pathology are characterized by more marked acidosis, more marked hypoxaemia in both the arterial and mixed venous blood, increased heart dimensions, such as those of the interventricular septum and the telediastolic diameter of the right ventricle, and from higher pulmonary arterial pressure values. The stepwise analysis of the most significant variables from the Student's t test suggested that RVI and IVS are the parameters most closely associated with the presence of RVH. Indeed, the following regression line was obtained:

$$RVAWT = 0.16 \times RVI + 0.31 \times IVS$$

where the estimated standard error turned out to be 1.1 mm with the significance level $P < 0.00001$ associated with the F test and the correlation coefficient, $R = 0.98$ (Fig. 4).

In a subsequent statistical calculation, the same variables were introduced without the echocardiographic values RVI and IVS: the variables mainly associated with the presence of RVH turned out to be pH and $P\overline{v}O_2$, according to the following regression line:

$$RVAWT = 146.9 - 18.5 \times pH - 0.1 \times P\overline{v}O_2$$

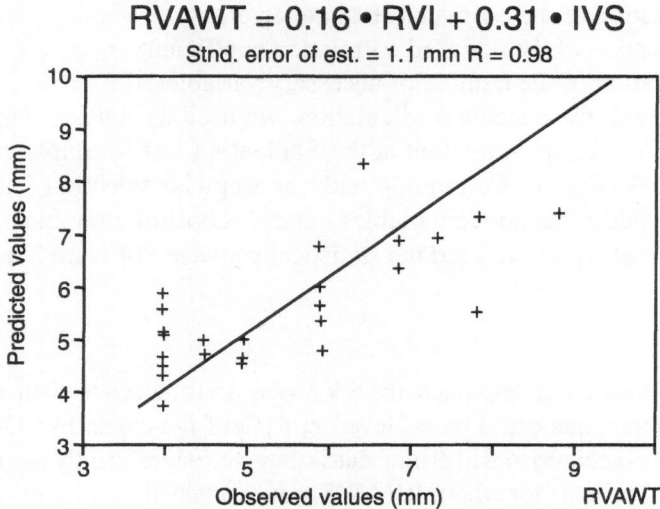

Fig. 4. Comparison between the observed and the predicted values of RVAWT according to the multiple regression analysis equation.

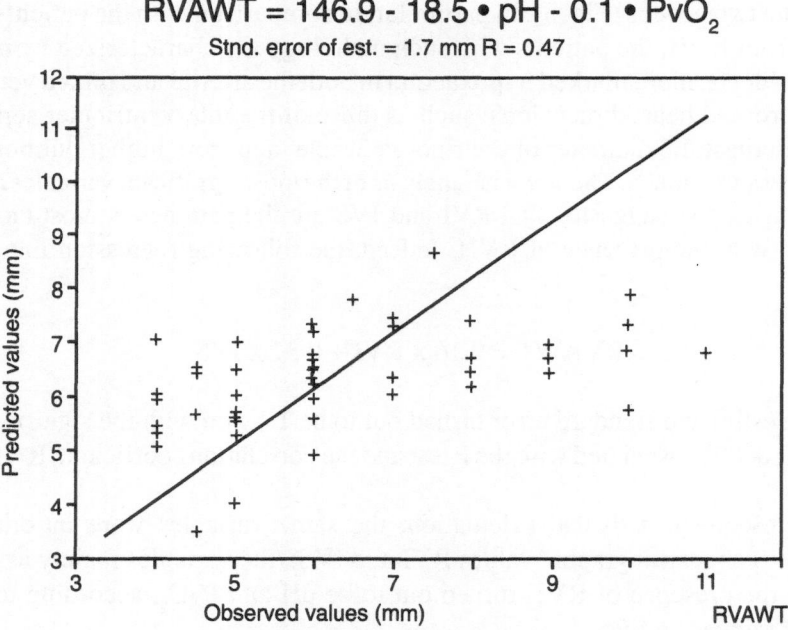

Fig. 5. Comparison between the observed and the predicted values of RVAWT according to the multiple regression analysis equation without echocardiographic values.

In this case, the estimated standard error was 1.7 mm and the correlation coefficient R = 0.47 (Fig. 5).

Discussion

Right ventricular hypertrophy is usually more difficult to detect and define as an entity, both from the clinical and anatomopathological viewpoint, than is the case for left ventricular hypertrophy.[8]

Nevertheless, in recent years, with the aid of echocardiography, several Authors have successfully studied the right heart and the largest pulmonary vessels.[7,8,9] Through the subcostal approach in COLD patients, echocardiographic images could be obtained which allow exact definition of the dimensions of the various heart structures.[10,11]

Moreover, according to additional reports, echocardiographic measurements of the right ventricular wall thickness can be very precise, they correlate well with the actual measurements of the right ventricular free wall at necropsy, and should, therefore, aid the physician in the diagnosis of RVH.[12,13]

Up to now, the mechanisms which during life concur in the determination of structural modifications of the right ventricle have been poorly understood. Thus, in the light of today's knowledge, it is difficult to define the factors fostering a "left ventriculization", that is the transformation of the right ventricle from volume to pressure pump with a thickening of its walls.[14]

According to the observations of some Authors[15], the main factors responsible for the onset of RVH in COLD are the extent and duration of pulmonary arterial hypertension, hypoxaemia and perhaps hypercarbia, physical activity, the exacerbation of respiratory diseases, the cardiac output, and the nutritional status.

Such aetiological agents could act through "mechanical" and "metabolic" mechanisms, such as the distension of myofibres and the variation of protein synthesis.[16]

Some authors affirm that right ventricular hypertrophy is a compensatory factor to pulmonary hypertension.[17] In our study, too, it can be observed that some haemodynamic factors, such as $\overline{PAP}$ and RVPSP, are significantly higher in the group of patients with RVH: thus, the concept is obviously very supportive of the existence of a cause-effect relationship between pressure overload and the onset of RVH.

However, the incidence of heart failure in COLD patients seems disproportionately high considering the mild to moderate degree of pulmonary hypertension typically found in this disease.[18] This stands in contrast to the less frequent occurrence of heart failure in patients with primary pulmonary hypertension in whom the increase in pulmonary vascular resistance is often so severe as to have produced syncope due to inadequate cardiac output and cerebral blood flow, yet peripheral oedema and other manifestations of heart failure are often absent. Thus, in addition to pulmonary hypertension, other factors may be operating in COLD patients to promote the occurrence of right ventricular hypertrophy. On the other hand, similar observations have been developed concerning the poor correlation between left ventricular hypertrophy and systemic arterial hypertension.[19,20,21]

As a matter of fact, according to our stepwise analysis, right ventricular hypertrophy is not associated mainly with haemodynamic variables but with the state of acidosis and hypoxaemia of the mixed venous blood. Widimsky et al.[22] showed that in adult male Wistar rats, at the beginning of their exposure to high altitude hypoxia, right ventricular hypertrophy could already be seen with focal necrotic lesions without, however, a significant change of the systolic right ventricular pressure. Moreover, Ishikawa et al.[23] found that in chronic cor pulmonale, a direct correlation exists between hypoxia and right ventricular fibre diameter but no correlation with hypercarbia or blood viscosity.

Furthermore, our data strengthen the results of the research performed by Kawakami et al.[24] who observed how arterial and mixed venous oxygenation are the main factors influencing the prognosis of COLD.

These as well as our data suggest the hypothesis that the mean tissue oxygen tension, which can be approximated from mixed venous oxygen tension[25], is one of the main factors concurring in the onset of right ventricular hypertrophy and, thus, accelerating the coming of right heart failure. The fact that, in the natural history of COLD, the onset of right ventricular hypertrophy occurs before the onset of heart failure is suggested also by some Authors who observed how the right ventricle in COLD tends first to dilate and then, in the most advanced phase, to hypertrophy[26]; this is different from what happens to the left ventricle subject to systemic arterial hypertension, which usually experiences concentric hypertrophy and, only subsequently, dilation. To confirm the above, in our study, we observed that the telediastolic diameter of the right ventricle in the patients with right ventricular hypertrophy increased in comparison with that of the group of patients without right ventricular hypertrophy. Moreover, our study showed that the thickening of the right ventricular anterior wall is also associated with the hypertrophy of the interventricular septum, though this structure is considered to mainly belong to the left ventricle.

These data reflect the responsiveness of the interventricular septum to the stimuli determining right ventricular hypertrophy. Our observation agrees with the results obtained by Ishikawa et al.[23] who demonstrated that in pure right ventricular hypertrophy secondary to pulmonary heart disease, not only the mean diameter of right ventricular fibres increases but also that of the interventricular septum, the latter being even larger than left ventricular fibres.

From our study, we may thus conclude that pulmonary hypertension in COLD cannot be considered as the main determining factor of RVH: a number of factors, such as the degree of tissue oxygenation and blood acidosis, seem to play a major role in the determination of structural modifications of the right ventricle.

References

1. McFadden E.R., Braunwald E.: Cor pulmonale, in E. Braunwald (Ed.): *Heart diseases*, Philadelphia Saunders Company, 1988; 1602
2. Fishman A.P.: Cor pulmonale, in Fishman A.P. (Ed.): *Pulmonary disease and disorders*, New York, McGraw-Hill book Co.:, 1980; 853
3. Bishop J.M., Csukas M.: Combined use of non-invasive techniques to predict pulmonary arterial pressure in chronic respiratory disease. Thorax 1989; 44:85-96
4. Denolin H.: Non-invasive diagnosis of pulmonary hypertension: a World Health Organization study. Herz 1986; 11:142-146
5. WHO: Nomenclature and definition in respiratory physiology and clinical aspects of chronic lung disease. Bull. Physiopath. Resp. 1975; 11:937
6. Bertoli L., Mantero A., Alpago R., Graziina A., Tamponi M., Pezzano A.: Value of two-dimensional echocardiography in the identification of pulmonary hypertrophy in chronic obstructive lung disease. Respiration 1989; 55: 193-201
7. Weiman A.E., *Cross-sectional echocardiography*, Philadelphia, Lea and Febiger, 1982; 382-395
8. Foale R., Nihoyannopoulos, McKenna W., Lienebenne A., Uadazdim A., Rowland E., Smith G.: Echocardiographic measurement of the normal adult right ventricle: Br. Heart J. 1986; 56:33
9. Bertoli L., Mantero A., Lo Cicero S., Alpago R., Rizzato G., Belli C.: Usefulness of two-dimensional echocardiography in the assessment of right heart in chronic obstructive lung disease. Prog. Respir. Res. 1985; 20:91-100
10. Danchin N., Cornette A., Henriquez A., Godenir J.P., Ethevenot G., Polu J.M., Sadoul P.: Two-dimensional echocardiographic assessment of the right ventricle in patients with chronic obstructive lung disease. Chest 1987; 92:229-233
11. Zenker G., Forche G., Harnoncourt K.: Two-dimensional echocardiography using a subcostal approach in patients with COPD. Chest 1985; 88:722-725
12. Prakash R.: Determination of right ventricular wall thickness in systole and diastole. Echocardiographic and necropsy correlation in 32 patients. Br. Heart J. 1978; 40:1257
14. Rahlf G., Schumacher W., Lenner C.T.: Quantitative anatomische Untersuchungen bei cor pulmonale chronicum, in Daum S., *Cor pulmonale chronicum*, Munich 1977; 63
15. Morpurgo M., Salviotti M.: La risposta del cuore all'ipertensione polmonare precapillare. Medicina Toracica 1983; 3:183-189
16. Hect A.: *Einfuehrung in experimentelle Grundlagen moderner Herzmuskelpathologie*, Jena, G. Vischer 1970; 586
17. Howard P.: Aetiological factors in hypoxic cor pulmonale. Progr. Resp. Res. 1985; 20:49-54
18. Rubin L.J.: Pulmonary hypertension secondary to lung disease. In: Weir E.K., Reeves J.T. (Eds.) *Pulmonary hypertension*. Mount Kisko, New York, Futura Publishing Company Inc. 1984; 291
19. Frohlich E.D., Tarazi R.C.: Is arterial pressure the sole factor responsible for hypertensive cardiac hypertrophy? Am. J. Cardiol. 1979; 44:959-963
20. Abi-Samura S., Fourd S.M., Tarazi R.C.: Determinants of left ventricular hypertrophy and function in hypertensive patients. Am. J. Med., 1983; 75 suppl. 3A:26-33
21. Drayer J.I.M., Weber M.A., De-Jaudig J.L.: Blood pressure as a determinant of cardiac left ventricular muscular mass. Arch. Int. Med. 1983; 143:90-92
22. Widimsky J., Urbanova D., Ressl J., Ostadal B., Pelouch V., Prochazka J.: Effect of intermittent altitude hypoxia on the myocardium and lesser circulation in the rat. Cardiovasc. Res. 1973; 7:798-808

76

23. Ishikawa S., Fattal G.A., Papiewicz J., Wyatt J.P.: Functional morphometry of myocardial fibers in cor pulmonale. Am. Rev. Resp. Dis. 1972; 105:358-367
24. Kawakami Y., Fishi F., Yamamoto H., Miyamoto K.: Relation of oxygen delivery, mixed venous oxygenation and pulmonary hemodynamics to prognosis in chronic obstructive pulmonary disease. N. Eng. J. Med. 1983; 308:1045-1049
25. Tenney S.M., Mithoefer J.C.: The relationship of mixed venous oxygenation to oxygen transport with special reference to adaptations to high altitude and pulmonary disease. Am. Rev. Respir. Dis. 1982; 135:474-479
26. Bertoli L., Rizzato G., Sala G., Merlini R., Lo Cicero S., Pezzano A.: Echocardiographic and hemodynamic assessment of right heart impairment in chronic obstructive lung disease. Respiration 1983; 44:282-288

Right Ventricular Function

7. Evaluation of Right Heart Failure: Controversies in Definitions and Methods of Evaluation

M. Morpurgo[1], V. Ježek[2]

1. Department of Cardiology, S. Carlo Borromeo Hospital, Milan, Italy
2. Institute of Physiological Regulations, Bulovka Hospital, Prague, Czechoslovakia

Characteristics of the Right Ventricle

The main function of the right ventricle (RV) is to maintain pressure in the very distensible venous system at a low level, i.e. significantly below the plasma oncotic pressure.[1,2] When the RV does not serve this function adequately, severe peripheral venous congestion and oedema supervene. The normal RV has been said to be more of a conduit than a pump.[3] It is the ability of the RV to generate the required stroke volume sufficient to maintain adequate cardiac output (volume pump), rather than its ability to generate pressure (pressure pump), that characterizes the function of the RV.

A better understanding of RV function has been hindered firstly by the perception that under many circumstances the contractile performance of the RV is haemodynamically unimportant. Additional work has demonstrated, however, that in the presence of haemodynamic stress, such as an elevated RV preload or afterload or coexistent left ventricular (LV) dysfunction, the depressed function of the injured RV does become important. Under such conditions, the amount of work generated by the RV is not sufficient to propel blood through the pulmonary circulation to maintain LV filling for adequate LV performance.[4] Baker et al.[5] observed that the RV ejection fraction at rest is more predictive of exercise capacity than LV ejection fraction in patients with chronic LV failure and demonstrated a clinically significant role of RV function in LV failure.

Furthermore, there is evidence that the RV may be more efficient than the left in terms of energetics: the normal RV may be converting more of the potential energy stored in its walls at maximum pressure into external mechanical work.[6]

The intact RV demonstrates the same length-dependent properties and the afterload independence of the contractile performance observed in the LV, so that RV and LV contractile performance may be perceived as fundamentally similar from the standpoint of muscle mechanisms.[4] Recent studies, however, confirm that identical changes in systolic pressure effect greater changes in systolic performance for the RV than for the LV.[7] Apparent differences in RV and LV function can be attributed to a variety of differences in extrinsic factors, such as lower impedance of pulmonary versus systemic circulation and relatively greater constraining effect of the pericardium on the RV.[4]

Many studies have shown that the anatomic bonds linking the two ventricles apparently influence their physiology as well, and create what eloquently has been defined as "cross-talk" between them.[8]

For instance, an increase in RV diastolic pressure will produce a concomitant rise in LV diastolic pressure and a decrease in LV dP/dt. In turn, RV is altered not only by the interplay with the LV, but also by at least four additional factors (Table I).

Table I. Factors influencing RV function

1. Influence of pericardium;
2. Effect of intrathoracic pressure;
3. Position and the motion of the interventricular septum;
4. Peculiar nature of the RV contractile arrangement, apparently due to the RV embryologic development.

Embryologic development is characterized by the evolution of two separate RV components to function in an integrated manner as the sinus (inflow) and conus (outflow) regions.[8] As pointed out by Foëx,[9] the outflow tract of the RV is anatomically different from the main portion of the RV; the internal surface of inflow and outflow tracts have contrasting topography. In the early phase of systole the inflow tract contracts while the outflow tract dilates;[3] the inflow tracts starts to relax earlier than the outflow tract. As shown by Zwissler et al.,[10] acute pulmonary microembolism in dog compromises the local RV function in the outflow tract, whereas the inflow tract is not affected. This could explain the limited diagnostic contribution of many noninvasive and invasive tools to the assessment of RV dysfunction, and stresses the importance of noninvasive methods developed in order to detect regional RV contraction abnormalities.[69]

From RV Hypertension to RV Dysfunction

The cardiac consequences of chronic pulmonary hypertension (PH), whatever its aetiology, are RV hypertrophy and/or dilatation and RV failure. Traditionally a distinction is made between a concentric and an eccentric type of hypertrophy, the latter most frequently associated with ventricular dilatation.

One cannot ignore, however, Horan's[11] conclusion that RV hypertrophy, i.e. increased RV free wall mass, and RV dilatation, i.e. increased free wall area, cannot be dissociated even at autopsy and can be properly referred to as one entity: RV enlargement.

On the other hand, RV enlargement has been used in the past to define the so-called "cor pulmonale".[12] It is possible that, as in systemic hypertension, the haemodynamic profile of the patient in terms of cardiac output, vascular resistance and arterial Windkessel properties, may determine the type of hypertrophy (concentric, eccentric; appropriate, inappropriate) that develops. Remodelling is much more important in the RV than in the LV and it signifies transformation from volume pump to pressure pump.

Chronic pressure overload hypertrophy may be viewed[13] as a beneficial adaptation that allows the ventricle to sustain increased work with the preservation of normal systolic wall stress and systolic shortening, and which may result in the performance of increased work with an improved metabolic and mechanical efficiency. In many instances, however, the price that is paid for these benefits is the development of heart failure due to diastolic dysfunction. In fact, pressure overload hypertrophy results in progressive impairment in diastolic distensibility of the ventricle, manifested as a substantial increase in ventricular filling pressure relative to diastolic volume.

The RV can maintain its function against a pressure overload provided LV and RV perfusion is maintained.[14] Pulmonary hypertension can be expected to increase coronary arterial resistance and thereby to decrease coronary arterial flow.[15] Actually, in patients with moderate to severe hypoxaemia due to chronic respiratory failure studied by Moret et al[16] the coronary arterial blood flow was found to be normal.

In 1971 Baroldi[17] presented data suggesting increased coronary artery size in "cor pulmonale"; however the correlation between coronary artery size and RV mass is poor according to Murphy's experience.[18]

The point is still controversial. Many pathological types of cardiac hypertrophy, particularly pressure-induced cardiac hypertrophy, are associated with a decrease in the cross-sectional area of the coronary vascular bed.[19] More data are needed before this "ischaemic" interpretation can be applied to patients with RV hypertrophy secondary to chronic lung disease.

On the subcellular level, the development of RV hypertrophy can be divided into three stages. In the first stage there is an increase in energy production, calcium accumulation and protein synthesis. In the second stage a stable state of cardiac hyperfunction is maintained. Finally, the third stage is characterized by gradual exhaustion of the ventricle.[20]

From RV Dysfunction to RV Failure

Major determinants of ventricular performance are: preload, afterload, contractility and heart rate.[21]

Preload is the passive force per cross-sectional area present in muscle fibre bundles before they contract.[22] Alterations in preload, operating through changes in end-diastolic dimensions, serve as important determinants of ventricular performance and provide the basis of end-diastolic pressure/stroke volume curves.[23] In clinical situations end-diastolic ventricular diameter, end-diastolic volume, end-diastolic ventricular pressure and right atrial pressure have been used to calculate the preloading of the RV.

Afterload is the instantaneous myocardial tension achieved during active contraction.[7] It is directly related to intracavitary pressure and to internal ventricular dimension, and inversely related to ventricular wall thickness. The pulmonary input impedance as well as the viscous and inertial properties of the blood contribute to the stress maintained in the ventricular wall during ejection. Afterload is never constant during ejection, but continually declines as ventricular volume and midwall radius decrease.[23]

Contractility measures the ability of the heart muscle to do stroke work independently of changes in initial fibre length.[22] Although contractility is the major determinant of cardiac performance, the term "ventricular contractility" has a different connotation from the term "ventricular performance"; it is useful to identify a change in contractility as an alteration in cardiac function that is independent of changes in ventricular performance, such as those caused by alterations in either preload, afterload or both.[23]

Certain loading conditions can produce failure of the ventricle as a pump in the absence of depression of myocardial contractility. On the other hand, depressed myocardial contractility may be masked by favourable loading conditions, resulting in no impairment of ventricular pump function.[4]

Several studies have recently emphasized the distinction between systolic and diastolic dysfunction. In diastolic dysfunction the ejection fraction (EF) at rest is within normal limits, but the rate of early ventricular filling is decreased.[24] Because of their different load dependence and different therapeutic range it is important to recognize the independent contribution of systolic and diastolic dysfunction in heart failure: a vertical displacement of the diastolic pressure/volume loop is associated with a reduced therapeutic range.[25]

What is "heart failure"? The physiologist regards the heart as failing when the contractility of the ventricle or the cardiac output fall outside the statistically defined normal range. The clinician regards his patient as having heart failure when there are symptoms or signs attributable to inadequate cardiac performance.[26]

According to Strobeck and Sonnenblick[23] the syndrome of heart failure may be considered in relation to two conditions.

The first is "myocardial failure", either diffuse or segmental, characterized by a decrease in speed and force of muscle contraction; when the amount of myocardial depression is great enough, it is translated into a decrease in the reserves of pump function and ultimately into pump failure.

The second condition is "congestive failure" which reflects systemic responses to an inadequate pump, characterized by augmented sympathetic nervous system activity, renal vasoconstriction and activation of the renin-angiotensin system. It brings about the necessity to include not only cardiac and circulatory function but also the renal and humoral mechanisms of compensation. The complex view on the topic could explain the discrepancies between the clinical picture of so-called "congestive right heart failure" and the wide spectrum of isolated haemodynamic findings in the same patient.

Myocardial failure always produces heart failure, but the converse is not necessarily the case, since a number of conditions in which the heart is suddenly overloaded can produce heart failure in the presence of normal myocardial function. Heart failure, in turn, always produces circulatory failure, but again the converse is not always true, since a variety of noncardiac situations can produce circulatory failure when cardiac function is normal or moderately impaired.[27]

The heart and the peripheral vasculature are linked very closely: one can influence the other in the context of physiological regulations or in the adaption to a pathological situation. The most recent progress in the field of cardiac failure derive from the concept of an interaction between centre and periphery.[28,29]

The dilated heart in failure is quite unable to "help itself" and is largely at the mercy of the peripheral circulatory reflexes for its further survival or ultimate demise.[30]

The situation in chronic obstructive lung disease could be slightly different: the cardiac output has been found normal by the majority of Authors even in patients with congestive failure. It can explain the normal values of oxygen tissue delivery despite an arterial hypoxaemia in these cases.

Many different adjectives have been added to the term "heart failure" in order to identify particular forms of disease or distinguish between different entities (right and left, forward or backward, systolic and diastolic). One can image a "latent" heart failure in which the muscle function is abnormal but the pump is still able to ensure an adequate output; and a "manifest" heart failure when myocardial function is so deeply altered that it cannot yield an adequate output.

The diagnosis of the initial setting is determined by the signs of the underlying disease (this is just the case in chronic lung disease) or by the consequences of compensatory mechanisms.[31] In the clinical sense, incipient right heart failure must be looked upon as a state where manifestations of decompensation appear during exposure to circulatory stress, such as physical strain and/or respiratory infectious disease.[32]

The distinction between right and left ventricular failure may be valid for the identification of the section of the heart primarily affected, but not from the functional standpoint, since the cardiac function is the product of the contribution of two sections, and in heart failure both ventricles are involved.[28]

Assessment of RV Enlargement

Whereas the LV has a fairly simple geometric shape and can be analysed with rather straightforward mathematical manipulations, the RV is an "amorphous object" that often defies simple geometrical analysis.[8] The heavy RV trabeculation contributes to the inaccuracy of geometric volume estimation and in any projection some overlap exists between the RV and other cardiac chambers. Furthermore, the RV tends to the alter its contour in the presence of pathological conditions.[33,34] In Kirch's[35] classical description of so-called "cor pulmonale" the shape of the heart often changes before any variation in wall thickness and weight of the RV occurs (Table II).

Table II. Noninvasive methods for the assessment of RV enlargement

---

- Electrocardiography and vectorcardiography
- M-mode and 2D-echocardiography
- Myocardial perfusion imaging with Thallium 201
- Magnetic resonance imaging (MRI)

The diagnostic contribution of different methods varies according to the aetiology of PH and RV enlargement.[36] Generally speaking, changes in wall thickness and in cavity dimensions of the RV are more pronounced when PH is due to thromboembolic disease or is apparently unexplained (so-called "primary" PH) than when it is due to chronic lung disease.

Since no single ECG criterion or combination of scalar and vectorial criteria is satisfactory for identification of RV hypertrophy in patients with chronic lung disease, also in our personal experience[37,38], and since we do not have personal data concerning myocardial perfusion scintigraphy and MRI, we shall limit our discussion to echocardiography.

M-mode and 2D-echocardiography are suitable for measurements of: 1. RV free wall thickness; 2. RV end-diastolic dimension; 3. diameter of the pulmonary artery. The presence of RV hypertrophy can be assessed from measurements of RV wall thickness and some correlations between measurements and autopsy data have been reported. However, it is often difficult to differentiate true RV wall from surrounding structures and the correlation between RV weight and RV wall thickness measured at autopsy has been found to be poor.[39,40] RV diastolic diameter as an isolated measurement or, better, as an index considering body surface area or LV end-diastolic diameter is a useful screening tool for the presence of RV enlargement. RV end-diastolic dimensions are higher in patients with previous episodes of RV failure;[41] these measurements may also be useful to assess the effect of therapy. Unfortunately, in patients with COPD echocardiography may be adequately performed in a limited percentage of cases.

Assessment of RV Dysfunction

In order to correctly evaluate the RV function one has to keep in mind that:
1. the right heart is a continuously changing entity in terms of pressure, flow and shape;
2. the RV ejects blood into a vascular bed submitted to continuous changes in dimensions and geometry;
3. between the RV and the pulmonary vessel bed there is a continuous interplay whereby the one influences the other and vice versa[42];
4. the RV is continuously assisted by the LV, having in common the stiff pericardial sac.

Furthermore, in the quantitative assessment of RV performance we must take into account the dissociation of RV pump function from myocardial contractility. The dependence of a variety of haemodynamic measurements on ventricular pump performance rather than on contractility has impaired most previous attempts to quantitate RV function. Moreover, function has been frequently described by indices used to quantitate LV performance, namely pressure derived indices and ejection fraction, that may not be sufficiently sensitive or accurate indicators of intrinsic RV contractile performance[4] (Tables III, IV).

Table III. Right ventricle *versus* left ventricle

- Complex geometric shape
- Morphologic heterogeneity
- Lower impedance of pulmonary circulation
- More important remodelling
- Greater constraining effect of pericardium
- Greater effect of systolic pressure on systolic performance

---

Table IV. The main noninvasive diagnostic tools for the assessment of RV dysfunction

- Radioisotopic measurement of RV ejection fraction;
- Echocardiographic (mechanocardiographic)measurements of RV systolic and diastolic time intervals;
- Exercise testing

The most commonly employed parameter of RV systolic performance, i.e. the ejection fraction (EF) is more easily altered by changes in loading conditions in the normally thin-walled RV than in the LV, and loading factors must be considered before a depressed RVEF may be interpreted to reflect RV myocardial pathology.[33] Actually, a variety of factors other than the intrinsic contractility have a marked effect on RVEF: one of these is the presence of tricuspid regurgitation.[43] Furthermore, RVEF reaction to exercise is influenced not only by exercise-induced changes in afterload, but probably also changes in the right coronary artery patency.[4] The EF as measured is determined not only by the extent of myocardial fibre shortening, but by the changing relations of the ventricular wall thickness to cavity size. Torsion of the heart during systole and fibre disarray in pathological conditions may also introduce errors.[44] In conclusion, although characteristically reduced in severe PH, RVEF does not appear to be a good parameter to assess intrinsic RV contractility.[4]

Functional RV changes can be detected by echocardiography and Doppler echocardiography in terms of:

1. velocity of fibre shortening during ejection: this measurement depends on uniform contraction of the heart and is rarely utilized for the evaluation of RV function;[45]
2. acceleration time: besides the level of pulmonary artery pressure, changes in RV contractility were recently reported to influence the acceleration time, contributing to its observed relation with age;[46]
3. systolic time intervals;
4. behaviour of the interventricular septum (IVS).

The typical response of the RV to pressure overload is a prolongation of the RV pre-ejection time (PEP) and a shortening of ejection time (RVET). Unfortunately, RV systolic time intervals are affected by RV preload, heart rate, intraventricular conduction defects and the presence of tricuspid insufficiency. Furthermore, experimental data produced by our group[47,48] show that the respiratory cycle deeply affects not only the duration of RVPEP and RVET, but also the pattern of the systolic plateau of the RV pressure curve, these changes being particularly evident at the transition from inspiration to expiration.

The position, curvature and pattern of motion of the IVS were found useful in differential diagnosis of RV overload.[7] Normally the IVS moves leftward during ejection and rightward during diastolic filling. In RV volume overload this pattern is reversed with rightward movement during ejection and leftward motion during filling (so-called paradoxical motion). With RV pressure overload the septum tends to be displaced toward the LV, with reduction in LV septal free wall dimensions throughout the cardiac cycle (reversed "Bernheim effect").

Coming now to the more sophisticated and invasive methods for the evaluation of RV function, one of the most useful indices of performance has been the ventricular function curve. Although ventricular function curves do not provide a description of ventricular contractile function which is independent of vascular loading conditions[49], the ventricular pressure/volume (P/V) diagram provides us with a rich source of information regarding ventricular performance as a pump. Particularly useful in this analysis is the end-systolic P/V relation (ESPVR).

Three interventions can shift the ventricular function curve: changes in contractility, changes in afterload and changes in ventricular compliance. In turn, apparent compliance (passive P/V relation) of the ventricle is determined not only by the passive properties of the wall, but also by the interaction of all chambers that are located inside the pericardial sac.

As the Starling relation describes the interaction between preload and systolic performance, the ESPVR describes the interaction between afterload and systolic performance. The slope of this relation may be termed "ventricular systolic elastance".[7] Ventricular elastance and particularly its peak value (E_{max}) can be used to represent the intrinsic force generating capability of the heart, because of both its negligible sensitivity to external loading and its behaving in a predictable manner with variations in contractile state. An increase in RV systolic pressure and end-diastolic volume results in a decrease in V_d (volume axis intercept of the peak elastance) without any change in E_{max}. An increase or a decrease in E_{max} can be interpreted to represent an augmentation or a depression of contractile state, respectively.[50] It must be stressed, however, that the P/V diagrams remove the important dimension of time and there are data to show that the P/V relationship is not always linear, thus invalidating E_{max}.

In general the slope of ESPVR is considerably shallower (greater volume change for a given change in pressure) for the RV than for the LV. Effect of age and chronic overload on E_{es} (end-systolic volume) and V_o (volume intercept of ESPVR on unstressed ventricular volume) needs to be clarified (Table V).

For clinical purposes, end-ejection volume may be derived from radionuclide ventriculography as minimal systolic volume.[7] It must be pointed out, however, that in the RV ejection continues for some time after the end-systolic point because the blood has considerable inertia and will continue to flow against the low-impedance vascular system despite a reversed pressure gradient. As a result, end-systole and end-ejection do not occur simultaneously.[49]

Table V. Limits of P/V relation measurements

To obtain both E_{es} and V_o one needs at least two P/V loops with substantially different end-systolic pressure under a constant inotropic state (Fig.1): Knowing the ESPVR at a single ESPV condition does not adequately characterize RV function as this single point could be on any contractility line.[51] Another difficulty in humans concerns the accuracy of RV volume measurements.[52] Reasonable accurate RV volumes may be obtained from biplane cineangio views that use oblique projections[53], particularly cranial axial oblique projections.[54]

- Not always linear[71]
- Not independent of loading conditions[6]*
- Not independent of host size[49]
- Sensitive to changes in ventricular compliance[45]
- RV end-ejection and end-systole do not coincide[52]
- Difficulty of accurate measurement of RV volumes[52]
- Need of two or more P/V loops[51]

* The more different V_o is from zero, the more it will affect the afterload dependence of P/V ratio (B.A. Carabello, 1990)

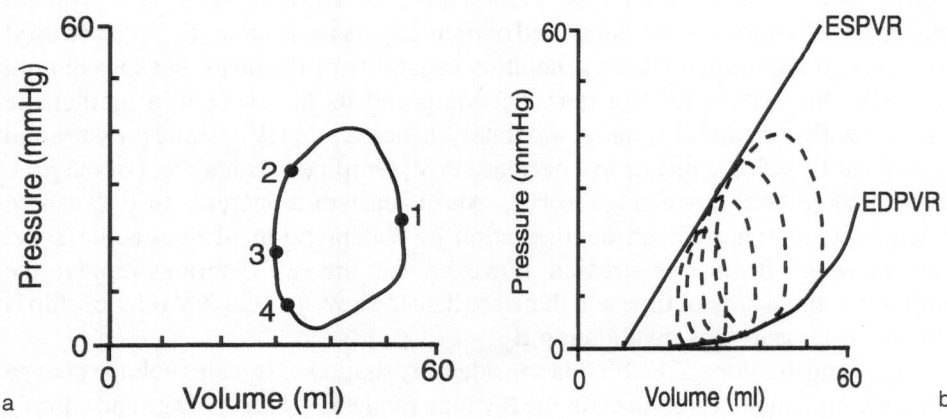

a

b

Fig. 1. Right ventricular P/V relationship (modified from W.L. Maugham and R.W. Oikawa[49]).
a. Right ventricular P/V loop recorded in the isolated heart preparation.
　　1 = starting point of ejection;
　　2 = peak RV volume elastance;
　　3 = end-ejection;
　　4 = starting point of filling.
b. The dashed P/V loops were recorded under steady-state conditions, ejecting against the same afterload, but with different filling pressures. The solid ESPVR and EDPVR lines connect the end-systolic and end-diastolic P/V points.

A new method for the assessment of RV function by intravenous digital angiography has been recently developed by Chappuis et al.[55]

The computer generates a time-volume curve showing RV volume changes during the entire cardiac cycle; RV pressure is simultaneously measured by a tip manometer. This sophisticated technique allows one to quantify RV systolic and diastolic function and to detect changes in RV function due to subtle alterations in loading conditions, like those induced by nitroglycerin.

The Frank-Starling relation can be represented by plotting stroke work (i.e. mean arterial pressure x stroke volume) against end-diastolic volume.[22] Expressing RV stroke work as a function of end-diastolic volume rather than end-diastolic pressure avoids the influence of factors that affect RV diastolic compliance, such as pericardial pressure and LV loading conditions.[4]

As for the isovolumetric phase indices, the dP/dt$_{max}$ used in the past for measuring acute directional changes in RV contractility in a given patient, for instance during isometric exercise,[56] has several limitations. This index is affected by end-diastolic pressure, arterial pressure and heart rate. Furthermore, since pressure development and rate of pressure development both depend on muscle mass and heart size, there is no easy way to normalize this index. Similarly, the calculations of isovolumetric V$_{max}$ met with several difficulties, including problems of measurement and assumption of muscle models. More important, there is a wide range in normals and considerable overlap with cardiac patients.[45]

What about the RV function at rest in patients with precapillary PH, particularly in PH due to chronic lung disease? From the clinical standpoint let us not forget that in 1891 Cardarelli[57] already wrote: "Emphysema, atelectasis, lung destruction, diffuse bronchitis, large pleural effusions and pneumothorax are able to create an obstacle in the pulmonary circulation and hence a hypersystole of the right ventricle".

In chronic RV pressure overload altered ejection fraction is often present, but abnormalities in RV contractility are generally absent.[7] In a group of patients with chronic lung disease Lewis and Christianson (personal communication) found that RVEF was reduced in 50% of cases, whereas cardiac index was normal in most cases. Analysis of the Starling relation showed that, with the same diastolic volume, stroke work was significantly greater in patients than in controls.

In the majority of COPD patients the systolic P/V ratio shifted to the left as compared to the normal curve, regardless of the level of afterload, indicating a RV "hyperfunction". These data have been recently confirmed by Burghuber and Bergmann[58] who observed that - despite a decreased RVEF - RV overall function (assessed by stroke volume index and cardiac index), as well as RV "contractility" (assessed by P/V relation) are well maintained in COPD patients, even in those with PH. These findings can explain the lack of effect of digitalis on RV performance in patients with COPD.[59]

In MacNee's experience[60,61] patients with COPD and past evidence of "cor pulmonale" who are studied when stable have relatively normal RV function in spite of the presence of PH at rest. Those who present acutely with "decompensated cor pulmonale" have depressed RV contractility. The observations mentioned above are in agreement with Widimsky's[32] statement: "In patients with cor pulmonale without clinically manifest right heart failure abnormal RV function which could be seen during exercise or even at rest is a rare phenomenon".

One should stress once more, however, that a possible impairment of RV contractility may be masked by compensatory changes in ventricular performance brought about by changes in loading conditions.[4]

Assessment of RV Function During Exercise (Table VI)

In healthy individuals the pulmonary vascular resistance (PVR) decreases passively on exercise in order to accommodate the increased cardiac output. The pathology of pulmonary vasculature does not allow the same response in patients with chronic lung disease and particularly in those with "vascular" forms of PH. The haemodynamic and cardiac response to exercise obviously varies according to the aetiology of PH, being different - for instance - in PH due to COPD and in PH secondary to pulmonary vascular disease, respectively (Table VI).

In patients with mild to moderate PH secondary chronic lung disease RVEF does not increase appropriately an aerobic exercise in response to the increased afterload. Conversely, both RV end-diastolic volume index and RV end-systolic volume index increase, suggesting that also in these patients one of the mechanisms by which stroke volume increases is the Frank-Starling mechanism.[62] In severe COPD patients Matthay and Berger[63] found that mean RVEF was less than 45% at rest and did not increase with exercise while subjects breathed room air, but improved significantly during exercise while patients breathed O_2 (2 l/min).

During symptom-limited exercise in COPD patients Morrison et al.[64] observed that the increase in cardiac output relative to VO_2 and VO_2 increase relative to work

Table VI. RV function during exercise

	Chronic lung disease	Pulmonary vascular disease
Cardiac output	normal	reduced
Oxygen delivery	normal	reduced
RV ejection fraction	reduced on room air normal on O_2	reduced
RV end-diastolic pressure	slightly increased	strongly increased

load were normal. Although COPD patients stop exercise at a far lower value of VO_2 and cardiac output than do normal subjects, the slope of this relation is comparable with that of normals. Whereas Morrison et al[15] found that COPD patients showed a smaller increase in heart rate (blunted heart rate response) in comparison with normal subjects during symptom-limited exercise, Light et al.[65] had noted that the pulse rate was elevated in COPD in relation to VO_2. Because the cardiac output was appropriate for VO_2, the stroke volume was diminished. Besides a RV dysfunction, chronic bronchodilator therapy and poor physical condition may have led to this relative tachycardia.

The discrepancy of some data reported in the literature may be due[6] to:

1. heterogeneity of the patients in different studies and even in the same study;
2. different methodological approaches;
3. the close interlinkage between cardiovascular and respiratory system.

As for this latter factor, the question whether cardiovascular or respiratory factors limit exercise in patients with COPD and PH seems to us irrelevant and will not be discussed here. Let us simply state that the interdependence of and linkage between different mechanisms during exercise was a stressed by Sir John Barcroft[67] in a book that contains three chapters entitled "Every adaptation is an integration".

In patients with pulmonary vascular disease without evidence of arterial O_2 desaturation during exercise the impairment to physical O_2 activity is predominantly a function of their compromised cardiac output response. The defect is a consequence of the inability to generate sufficient pulmonary blood flow to sustain LV filling. These patients do not benefit from regular exercise due to the dramatic increase in pressure load that confronts the RV.[6]

To conclude, let us formulate a few suggestions:

1. Avoid the term "contractility" when actually you are evaluating pump performance.
2. Consider that pump function may appear normal in presence of impaired contractility if loading conditions are favourable.
3. Do not apply to the RV measurements or indices simply because they were good for the left heart.
4. Consider RV function synthetically rather than in terms of separate measurements.

The synthetic approach should obviously start from the RV, but through a broader vision of the ventricular interdependence and of the cardiopulmonary unit, it should attain the dimension of the global cardiovascular unit or, even better, of the gas transport system, without which life could not exist.[68]

92

References

1. Furey S.A., Zieske H.A., Levy M.N.: The essential function of the right ventricle. Am. Heart J. 1984; 107:404-410
2. Gioffrè P.A., Gaspardone A., Pelliccia F.: Aspetti funzionali del ventricolo destro. Primary Cardiology 1987; 2:65-71
3. Oakley C.: Importance of right ventricular function in congestive heart failure. Am. J. Cardiol. 1988; 62:14A-19A
4. Morris J.M., Wechsler A.S.: Right ventricular function: the assessment of contractile performance. In: Fisk R.L., et al.(Eds.): *The Right Heart*, Philadelphia, Davis Co., 1987; 3-18
5. Baker B.J., Wilen M.M., Boyd C.M., Ha Dinh, Franciosa J.A.: Relation of right ventricular ejection fraction to exercise capacity in chronic left ventricular failure. Am. J. Cardiol. 1984; 54:596-599
6. Redington A.N., Gray H.H., Hodson M.E., Rigby M.L., Oldershaw P.J.: Characterization of the normal right ventricular pressure-volume relation by biplane angiography and simultaneous micromanometer pressure measurements. Br. Heart J. 1988; 59:23-30
7. Konstam M.A., Levine H.J.: Effects of afterload and preload on right ventricular systolic performance. In: Konstam M.A., Isner J.M. (Eds.) *The Right Ventricle*. Boston, Kluwer Acad. Publ. 1988; 17-35
8. Ferlinz J.: Right ventricular function in adult cardiovascular disease. Progr. Cardiovasc. Dis. 1982; 25:225-267
9. Foex P.: Right ventricular contraction. In: Vincent J.L., Suter P.M.(Eds.): *Cardiopulmonary Interactions in Acute Respiratory Failure*. Springer-Verlag, Berlin 1987; 72-80
10. Zwissler B., Forst H., Messmer K.: Influence of acute pulmonary embolism on local and global contractility of the canine right ventricle. Intern. Symposium Pulmonary Circulation V, Prague, (abstr.), 1989; 191
11. Horan L.G., Flowers N.C., Havelda C.J.: Relation between right ventricular mass and cavity size: an analysis of 1500 human hearts. Circulation 1981; 64:135-138
12. Ferrer M.I.: Cor pulmonale (pulmonary heart disease): present-day status. Am. Heart J. 1975; 89:657-664
13. Lorell B.H., Grossman W.: Cardiac hypertrophy: the consequences for diastole. JACC 1987; 9:1189-1193
14. Morrison D., Goldman S., Wright A.L., Henry R., Sorenson S., Caldwell J.H., Ritchie J.: The effect of pulmonary hypertension on systolic function of the right ventricle. Chest 1983; 84:250-257
15. Morrison D., Ackock K., Collins C.M., Goldman S., Caldwell J.H., Schwartz M.I.: Right ventricular dysfunction and exercise limitation of chronic obstructive pulmonary disease. JACC 1987; 9:1219-1229
16. Moret P.R., Boufas D., Fournet P.C.: Circulation coronaire et mètabolisme du myocarde dans le coeur pulmonaire chronique. Arch. Mal. Coeur 1969; 8:1168-1172
17. Baroldi G.: (personal communication)
18. Murphy M.L.: The pathology of the right heart in chronic hypertrophy and failure. In: Fisk R.L., (Ed.): *The Right Heart*. Philadelphia, Davis Co., 1987; 159-169
19. Marcus M.L., Harrison D.G., Chilian W.M., Koyanagi S., Inou T., Tomanek R.J., Martins J.B., Easthman C.L., Hiratzka L.F.: Alterations in the coronary circulation in hypertrophied ventricles. Circulation 1987; 75 (Suppl. 1):1-19
20. Meerson F.Z.: The myocardium in hyperfunction, hypertrophy and heart failure. Circ. Res. 1969; 25 (Suppl. 2):1

21. Green J.F.: *Fundamental Cardiovascular and Pulmonary Physiology*. Lea and Febiger, Philadelphia, 1987; 45-55

22. Goerke J., Mines A.H.: *Cardiovascular Physiology*: New York, Raven Press, 1988; 99-152

23. Strobeck J.E., Sonnenblick E.H.: Pathophysiology of heart failure: In: Levine H.J:, Gaasch W.H. (Eds.) *The ventricle*. Boston, Martinus Nijhoff Publ. 1985; 209-224

24. Poole-Wilson P.A.: The origin of symptoms in patients with chronic heart failure. Europ. Heart J. 1988; 9 (Suppl. H):49-53

25. Kramer W.: Kardiale und extrakardiale Parameter als Grundlage differential-therapeutischer Ueberlegungen bei Vor-und Nachlastsenkung. Z. Kardiol. 1988; 77 (Suppl. 5):87-96

26. Julian D.G.: *Cardiology*. London, Bailliere Tindall,1983; 9

27. Braunwald E.: Comment to Denolin H., et al.: The definition of heart failure. Europ. Heart J. 1983; 4:445-448

28. Guazzi M.: Lo scompenso cardiaco. Cardiologia 1983; 33 (Suppl. 1):275-283

29. Zelis R., Sinoway L.I., Musch T.I.: Why do patients with congestive heart failure stop exercising? JACC 1988; 12:359-361

30. Taylor S.H.: Cardiovascular consequences of heart failure. Europ. Heart J. 1988; 9 (Suppl. H):41-47

31. Denolin H.: Conclusion International Symposium "L'insufficienza cardiaca latente". Venezia 1977; 609-615

32. Widimsky J.: Latent cardiac insufficiency in chronic cor pulmonale: International Symposium "L'insufficienza cardiaca latente". Venezia 1977; 389-402

33. Konstam M.A., Pandian N.: Assessment of right ventricular function. In Konstam M.A., Isner J.M., (Eds.): *The Right Ventricle*. Boston, Kluwer Acad. Publ. 1988; 1-15

34. Dittrich H.C., Nicod P.H., Chow L.C., Chappuis F.P., Moser K.M., Peterson K.L.: Early changes of right geometry after pulmonary thromboendarterectomy. JACC 1988; 11:937-943

35. Kirch E.: Die pathologische Anatomie des Cor pulmonale. Verh. Dtsch.Ges. Kreislaufforsch1955; 21:163-181

36. Morpurgo M.: Non-invasive methods for the assessment of pulmonary arterial hypertension. Med. Torac. 1981; 3:263-268

37. Morpurgo M., Moccetti T.: The contribution of electrocardiography to the diagnosis of chronic cor pulmonale: a critical reappraisal. In: Daum S. (Ed.) *Cor pulmonale Chronicum*. München 1977; 286-298

38. Bottoni R., Mandelli V., Marzegalli M., Moccetti T., Morpurgo M.: Predittività dei criteri elettrocardiografici e vettrocardiografici nell'ipertensione arteriosa polmonare da bronco-pneumopatie croniche. G. Ital. Cardiol. 1979; 9:390-399

39. Mitchell R.S., Stanford R.E., Silvers G.W., Dart G.: The right ventricle in chronic airway obstruction: a clinico-pathologic study. Am. Rev. resp. Dis. 1976; 11:147-154

40. Murphy M.L.: The pathology of the right heart in chronic hypertrophy and failure. In: Fisk R.L. (Ed.) *The Right Heart* Philadelphia, Davis Co. 1987; 159-169

41. Danchin N., Cornette A., Henriquez A., Godenir J.P., Ethevenot G., Polu J.M., Sadoul P.: Two-dimensional echocardiographic assessment of the right ventricle in patients with chronic obstructive lung disease. Chest 1987; 92:229-233

42. Piene H.: Pulmonary arterial impedance and right ventricular function. Physiol. Rev. 1986; 66:606-652

43. Morrison D.A., Ovitt T., Hammersameister K.E.: Functional tricuspid regurgitation and right ventricular dysfunction in pulmonary hypertension. Am. J. Cardiol. 1988; 62:108-112

44. Altschule M.D.: Limited usefulness of the so-called ejection fraction measurement in clinical practice. Chest 1986; 90:134-135

94

45. Parmley W.W.: Mechanics of ventricular muscle. In: Levine H.J., Gaasch W.H. (Eds.): *The Ventricle*. Boston, Martinus Nijhoff Publ. 1985; 41-62
46. Vaska K., Sagar K., Wann L.S.: Pulmonary Doppler ultrasound depends on right ventricular inotropic state as well as pulmonary artery systolic pressure (abstr.). Circulation 1988; 78 (Suppl. 2):402
47. Rustici A., Fogari R., Grossoni M., Tommasini R., Ukmar G., Morpurgo M.: Influence of spontaneous respiration on right ventricular systolic time intervals and pulmonary arterial pressures in the dog. In: Daum S. (Eds.) *Interaction between heart and lung*. Thieme, Stuttgart, 1989; 18-24
48. Rustici A., Grossoni M., Ukmar G., Tommasini R., Morpurgo M.: Quali momenti del ciclo respiratorio influiscono maggiormente sulla dinamica del ventricolo destro? G. Ital. Cardiol. 1988; 18:1018-1024
49. Maughan W.L., Oikawa R.Y.: Right ventricular function. In: Scharf S.M., New York, M. Dekker 1989; 179-220
50. Weber K.T., Janicki J.S., Shroff S.J.: The heart as a mechanical pump. In: Weber K.T., Janicki J.S.(Eds.) *Cardiopulmonary Exercise Testing*. Philadelphia, Saunders 1986; 34-56
51. Albert R.K.: Assessment of right ventricular function. Chest 1988; 94:1123-1124
52. Sagawa R., Sunagawa K., Maughan W.L.: Ventricular end-systolic pressure-volume relations. In: Levine H.J., Gaasch W.H. (Eds.) *The ventricle*. Boston, Martinus Nijhoff Publ. 1985; 79-103
53. Duabert J.C., Descaves C., Langella B., Mabo P., de Place C.: La cinéangiographie seléctive du ventricule droit: technique, résultats et intérets pratiques. L'Information cardiologique 1988; 12:487-510
54. Pietras R.J., Kondos G.T., Kaplan D.: Quantitative validation of cineangiographic biplane axial oblique right ventricular volume measurement. Am. Heart J. 1987; 321-325
55. Chappuis E., Dorsaz P.A., Rutishauser W.: New method for the assessment of right ventricular function by intravenous digital angiography. First International Workshop on New Trend in Cardiovascular Therapy and technology, Genoa, 1989 (abstr.):25P
56. Pastorini C., Iannetti M., Marsano C., Caponnetto S.: Valutazione della funzione globale e della meccanica muscolare del ventricolo destro a riposo e durante lo sforzo isometrico in soggetti affetti da broncopneumopatia cronica ostruttiva senza segni di scompenso cardiaco. G. Emodinam. 1983; 3:73-80
57. Cardarelli A.: Le malattie nervose e funzionali del cuore. Napoli, C.Domenico Ed. 1891; 330-331
58. Burghuber O.C., Bergmann H.: Right-contractility in chronic obstructive pulmonary disease: a combined radionuclide and hemodynamic study. Respiration 1988; 53:1-12
59. Berglund E.: Hemodynamics of the right ventricle in chronic lung disease. Bull. Physiol. Resp. 1972; 8:1417-1422
60. MacNee W.: Right ventricular function in cor pulmonale. Cardiology 1988; 75 (suppl. 1):30-40
61. MacNee W., Wathen C.G., Flenley D.C., Muir A.D.: The effects of controlled oxygen therapy on ventricular function in patients with stable decompensated cor pulmonale. Am. Rev. Resp. Dis. 1988; 137:1289-1295
62. Loke J., Mahler D.A., Man S.F.P., Wiedemann H.P., Matthay R.A.: Exercise impairment in chronic obstructive pulmonary disease. Clin. Chest Med. 1984; 129-143
63. Matthay R.A., Berger H.J.: Noninvasive assessment of right and left ventricular function in acute and chronic respiratory failure. Crit. Care Med. 1983; 11:329-337
64. Morrison D.A., Adcock K., Collins C.M., Goldman S., Caldwell J.H., Schwartz M.I.: Right ventricular dysfunction and the exercise limitation of chronic obstructive pulmonary disease, JACC 1987; 9: 1219-1229
65. Light R.W., Mintz H.M., Linden G.S., Brown S.E.: Hemodynamics of patients with severe

chronic obstructive pulmonary disease during progressive upright exercise. Am. Rev. Res. Dis. 1984; 130:391-395

66. Morpurgo M., Denolin H.: The heart in pulmonary hypertension due to chronic lung disease. In: Wagenvoort C.A., Denolin H. (Eds.) *Pulmonary Circulation.* Amsterdam, Elsevier, 1989; 163-189

67. Barcroft J.: *Features in the Architecture of Physiological Function.* London, Cambridge University Press, 1934

68. Weber K.T., Janicki J.S.: Pulmonary hypertension. In Weber K.T., Janicki J.S. (Eds.) *Cardiopulmonary Exercise Testing.* Philadelphia, Saunders, 1986; 220-235

69. Wassermann K.: New concepts in assessing cardiovascular function. Circulation 1988; 78:1060-1071

70. Ratner S.J., Huang P.J., Friedman M.I., Pierson R.N.: Assessment of right ventricular anatomy and function by quantitative radionuclide ventriculography. JACC, 1989; 13:354-359

71. Noble M.I.M.: The pressure-volume relationship of the intact heart. In: H.E.D.J. ter Keurs, M.I.M. Noble (Eds.) *Starling's Law of the Heart Revisited.* Dordrecht, Kluwer Acad. Publ. 1988; 126

8. Clinical Diagnosis of Right Heart Failure in Chronic Obstructive Lung Disease

H. DENOLIN

Department of Cardiology, Saint-Pierre University Hospital, Brussels, Belgium

When considering the literature on right heart failure in chronic obstructive lung disease (COLD) we are faced immediately with problems of definitions.

The first definition is "cor pulmonale": for some authors cor pulmonale includes the right heart failure secondary to pulmonary disease; for others, and this is probably more correct, we should clinically distinguish pulmonary hypertension from cor pulmonale - the adaptive right ventricular enlargement - and from cor pulmonale with right heart failure. Another problem of definition is heart failure. Many definitions of heart failure were proposed, but there is finally no generally accepted definition. A few years ago, a working group of the European Society of Cardiology tried again to formulate a definition:[1]

Heart failure is the state of any heart disease in which, despite adequate ventricular filling, the heart's output is decreased or in which the heart is unable to pump blood at the rate adequate for satisfying the requirements of the tissues with function parameters remaining within normal limits.

The comments following this definition demonstrate that it is not an acceptable definition for some of our colleagues and, in any case, is probably more related to a deficiency of the arterial side of the circulation. For the venous side of the circulation, *heart failure denotes an inability of one or more chambers of the heart to accept and expel the venous return throughout the range of physiologic activity without alteration of normal circulatory haemodynamics.*[2] So, heart failure remains difficult to define, and many authors suggest using the term as a clinical description only.

The classic signs of right ventricular failure in COLD consist of engorgement of the great veins, including the jugular veins, liver enlargement and tenderness, ascites and oedema of the legs.[3,4]

These signs are the same as those described in any other cause of right heart failure. But are venous distension and oedema really related to right ventricular failure in COLD?

The question can be raised if we consider:

a. that in COLD pulmonary hypertension is generally of mild degree;
b. that cardiac output at rest is almost always within normal range, and the response to exercise is also normal;[5]
c. that several recent studies have concluded there is relatively normal right heart contractility in the majority of patients with COLD.[6-7]

This is a quotation from Rubin: *We have performed right heart catheterization in six patients referred to us with severe chronic obstructive lung disease, oedema and cor pulmonale only to find that haemodynamic measurements, both at rest and during exercise, were normal.*[8]

The conclusion of these observations could be that signs suggesting right ventricular failure may develop in patients with pulmonary hypertensive heart disease, even with a cardiac muscle performing normally as a contractile tissue, and that there is little evidence for true right ventricular failure in cor pulmonale.

But this is a negative conclusion. How can one explain the clinical signs like distension of the neck veins or oedema?

The venous distension can be explained by the excessive fall of intrathoracic pressure during inspiration and the collapse of the great veins at the thoracic inlet. Therefore, distended jugular veins may occur during inspiration without right ventricular failure.

What about oedema? Here again, the role of right heart failure is doubtful. The fact that in chronic lung disease oedema is not closely correlated with right ventricular hypertrophy, raised venous pressure or pulmonary hypertension was already suggested by several authors. For Campbell and Short[11], some or many patients with cor pulmonale and oedema may not pass through the final common pathway of pulmonary hypertension and right ventricular failure.

But what are the other possible causes of oedema to be considered? There are few observations, but most consistent is the fall in renal blood flow when oedema develops.[9] Hypoxaemia and hypercapnia would seem the most likely cause. There is a retention of sodium and water through renal mechanisms, predominantly the renin-angiotensin system and also a redistribution of intracellular water to the extracellular space[10]; any respiratory acidosis may be more important than right heart failure.[11-12] Fineberg et al. demonstrated that hypoxia in the presence of hypercapnia may contribute significantly to sodium retention and oedema by adversely affecting glomerular function.[13] A glomerular enlargement was demonstrated in cor pulmonale, related to the degree of hypoxaemia.[14] Redistribution may be caused by an increased requirements for extracellular cations to buffer respiratory acidosis.

In summary, peripheral oedema occurring in patients with chronic obstructive lung disease, formerly attributed to heart failure, is probably related in many cases to impaired renal function, but the mechanisms involved remain to be explained.

So the problem is not to recognize clinical signs of heart failure, but to decide if clinical signs are related to heart failure. The evaluation of heart failure should be established by other methods than clinical: this is important from the therapeutic point of view.

References

1. Denolin H., Kuhn H., Krayenbuehl H.P., Loogen F., Reale A.: The definition of heart failure. Eur. Heart J. 1983;4: 445
2. Friedberg C.K.: *Diseases of the heart.* Philadelphia, 3rd Edition, Saunders, 1966
3. White P.D.: *Heart Disease.* New York, 3rd Edition, Macmillan, 1945
4. Denolin H.: *Le diagnostic clinique du coeur pulmonaire chronique. Cor pulmonale chronicum.* München 1977; 283
5. Bishop J.M.: Does pulmonary arterial hypertension influence the prognosis in patients with chronic obstructive lung disease? Cor Vasa 1985; 27, 172
6. MacNee W: Right ventricular function in cor pulmonale. Cardiology, 1988; 75 (Suppl. 1),30
7. Biernacki W., Flenley D., Muir A.L., MacNee W.: Pulmonary hypertension and right ventricular function in patients with COPD. Chest 1988; 94, 1169
8. Rubin L.J.: Clinical evaluation. In: Rubin L.J. (Ed.): *Pulmonary heart disease.* Boston, M. Nijhoff, 1984
9. Richens J.M., Howard P.: Oedema in cor pulmonale. Clinical Science 1982; 62, 255
10. Howard P., Suggett A.J.: Cor pulmonale. In: Sleight P., Vann Jones, J. (Ed.) *Cardiology.* London, W.Heinemann, 1983
11. Campbell E.J.M., Short D.S.: The cause of oedema in "cor pulmonale". Lancet 1960; 1, 1184
12. Chiappini M.G., Manfellotto D., Gentile S., Darses N., Re M.A., Peruzzi G., Vulterini S.: Hydro-Saline retention in COLD patients with respiratory failure. Eur. J. Respir. Dis. 1986; 69 (Suppl. 146) 359
13. Fineberg N.S., Dowdeswell J.R.G., Burt R.W., Manfredi F.: Effect of hypoxemia on sodium and water excretion in chronic obstructive lung disease. Am. J. Med. 1985; 78, 87
14. Campbell J.L., Calverley P.M., Lamb D., Flenley D.: The renal glomerulus in hypoxic cor pulmonale. Thorax 1982; 37, 607

9. Cardiac Output in Chronic Lung Diseases

V. Ježek[1], E. Weitzenblum[2], F. Schrijen[3], J. Zielinski[4]

1. *Institute of Physiological Regulations, Czechoslovak Academy of Sciences, Prague, Czechoslovakia*
2. *Pulmonary Function Laboratory, University Hospital, Pavillon Laennec, Strasbourg, France*
3. *INSERM, Unit 14, Nancy, France*
4. *Department of Respiratory Medicine, Institute of Tuberculosis, University Hospital, Warsaw, Poland*

Introduction

It was postulated at the very beginning of the catheterization era that cardiac output (CO) in chronic lung disease (CLD) is elevated[1]; decompensated cor pulmonale was included within so-called *high output failure*.[2] Nevertheless, most Authors did not confirm these findings, during following decades which could have been influenced by the imperfect methods of that era.[3] They found a normal CO in most instances.[4-6]

Harris and Heath[7] summarized the results of several studies and they concluded that CO is almost the same in patients with and without cardiac failure.[8-13] This finding contrasted with the substantially lower CO in right heart failure of cardiac origin.[4,14,15]

Moreover, most authors found that CO increases normally, i.e. proportionally to oxygen consumption, in CLD both with and without cardiac failure.[16-21]

As for the longitudinal follow-up, Burrows et al.[22] and Filley et al.[23] noted a stepwise decrease of CO during the development of cardiac failure. It was not confirmed by others[24] and no consistent change of CO has been found during long-term evaluation of patients with chronic obstructive lung disease (COLD).[25-27]

All these data concern the haemodynamics in COLD. The situation in other chronic lung diseases (except the so-called primary pulmonary hypertension) has seldom been studied.

Our intention was to complete these data also in patients with chronic restrictive lung disease (CRLD) and to compare them with cardiac patients. A further goal of our study was to assess the haemodynamics shortly before death in these patient categories.

Patients and Methods

a. Haemodynamics at rest and during exercise

The subgroup of COLD consists of patients from our previous studies[28-31] and it comprises 54 patients always free from cardiac failure and 19 patients examined with clinical signs of failure (leg oedema, hepatomegaly and distended neck veins). The criteria of COLD are given in the original papers.

The subgroup of CRLD includes 28 patients always free from right heart failure and 8 patients examined in clinical cardiac failure. The diagnosis in all subjects was diffuse interstitial lung fibrosis; it was confirmed by the lung biopsy in 24 subjects and by typical functional examination in the remaining ones. The exercise was performed on a bicycle ergometer in the supine position, speed 50 cycles/min, work load from 20 to 40 Watts/min during 5-6 minutes.

The results were compared with 34 cardiac patients examined in the same manner; their diagnosis was ischaemic heart disease in 18 and valvular heart disease (aortic or mitral, without dominant stenosis) in the remaining 16 cases. The haemodynamic response to exercise we also compared with the response of healthy volunteers.[35]

b. Preterminal haemodynamics

This group of patients differs from all preceding ones. It was recently collected from all participating centres (Prague, Strasbourg, Nancy, Warsaw). It included:

- 16 patients with COLD, 12 of them with 2 catheterizations;
- 12 patients with CRLD, 9 of them with 2 catheterizations;
- 16 cardiac patients (ischaemic or valvular), 9 of them with 2 catheterizations.

Inclusion criteria for this part of the study were as follows:

1. The last catheterization should be performed not longer than 3 months before death.
2. The condition of patients between the last catheterization and death should be stable. All patients with lung embolism, acute exacerbation of respiratory insufficiency, myocardial infarction and nonspecified sudden death were excluded.
3. The patients should preferably have had another catheterization before in order to assess the haemodynamic evolution.

This condition was fulfilled in 30 patients and the interval between both catheterizations was 2.1±2.0 years. The technique of catheterization was the same in all participating centres. All values were calculated according to usual formulae.[32]

The right ventricular work was expressed as a product of CO and the difference between the mean pulmonary arterial and mean right atrial pressures.

The oxygen tissue delivery (OD) was calculated as a product of CO and the oxygen content in arterial blood; OD divided by the oxygen consumption was classified as oxygen delivery index (ODI).

The results were compared with normal values obtained in the Prague centre (Table I).

The statistical analysis was performed by the calculation of variance and by the least-squares correlation coefficients.[33,34]

Table I. Normal values obtained in 35 subjects without proven pulmonary or cardiovascular disease

Value	Mean	SD
Age (years)	32.900	12.600
PaO_2 (mmHg)	81.600	6.700
SaO_2 (%)	95.800	1.400
$\overline{P}_{ra}$ (mmHg)	3.200	2.300
$\overline{P}_{pa}$ (mmHg)	14.200	2.900
$\overline{P}_{w}$ (mmHg)	7.600	2.500
$\dot{Q}$ (1 min^{-1} m^{-2})	3.010	0.470
SV (ml m^{-2})	39.500	7.900
PVR (dyn s cm^{-5})	99.500	39.700
W_R (W m^{-2})	0.073	0.019
RVSW (mJ m^{-2})	57.500	15.900
O_2D (ml min^{-1} m^{-2})	540.000	83.000
ODI	4.060	0.430

PaO_2 = arterial oxygen tension;
SaO_2 = arterial oxygen saturation;
$\overline{P}_{ra}$ = mean right atrial pressure;
$\overline{P}_{pa}$ = mean pulmonary arterial pressure;
$\overline{P}_{w}$ = mean pulmonary wedge pressure;
$\dot{Q}$ = cardiac index;
SV = stroke volume index;
PVR = pulmonary vascular resistance;
W_R = right ventricular work;
RVSW = right ventricular stroke work;
O_2D = oxygen tissue delivery;
ODI = oxygen delivery index.

Table II. Hemodynamics at rest and during exercise in three subgroups of patients

Value		COLD Comp. (54)	Decomp. (19)	CLRD Comp. (28)	Decomp. (8)	Cardiac patiens (34)
$\overline{P}_{ra}$	R	6.20± 3.00	10.70±3.30	2.90±2.90	4.10±2.80	5.10±4.20
(mmHg)	E	7.70±3.50	18.90±6.90	0.90±4.20	10.30±2.90	11.40±6.70
$\dot{Q}$	R	3.29±0.85	3.31±1.40	2.97±0.57	2.73±0.64	2.33±0.32
(1 min^{-1} m^{-2})	E	5.68±1.55	5.64±1.70	5.11±1.33	4.63±0.93	3.50±0.85
SV	R	40.10±10.00	37.60±10.50	36.80±5.70	31.80±5.00	33.50±5.3
(ml m^{-2})	E	53.10±13.50	50.40±13.50	45.00±11.80	39.90±6.30	33.10±9.6
HR	R	81.00±10.00	89.00±12.00	81.00±12.00	86.00±14.00	70.00±12.00
(min^{-1})	E	107.00±14.00	114.00±12.00	116.00±19.00	116.00±14.00	110.00±23.00
$\dot{V}O_2$	R	156.00±15.00	152.00±14.00	130.00±19.00	124.00±14.00	124.00±21.00
(ml min^{-1} m^{-2})	E	416.00±77.00	432.00±83.00	310.00±86.00	290.00±55.00	345.00±64.00
RVSW	R	76.00±30.00	98.00±50.00	72.00±19.00	103.00±60.00	106.00±49.00
(ml m^{-2})	E	176.00±61.00	118.00±87.00	155.00±53.00	207.00±78.00	192.00±99.00
OD	R	602.00±105.00	610.00±111.00	545.00±94.00	518.00±97.00	435.00±66.00
(ml min^{-1} m^{-2})	E	1037.00±216.00	965.00±201.00	887.00±190.00	793.00±124.00	643.00±45.00
ODI	R	3.81±0.58	4.04±0.66	4.21±0.52	4.18±0.62	3.58±0.49
	E	2.42±0.44	2.23±0.38	2.93±0.52	2.84±0.70	1.89±0.24

R = rest;
E = exercise;
COLD = chronic obstructive lung disease;
CRLD = chronic restrictive lung disease;
HR = heart rate.
Remaining abbreviations are the same as in Table I

Results

1. Adaptation to exercise in individual groups of patients
These results are summarized in Table II.
COLD without right heart failure (RHF): insignificant change of right atrial pressure is associated with appropriate rise of stroke volume and the increase of CO is proportional to the rise of oxygen consumption (Fig. 1). The oxygen tissue delivery is normal and it rises adequately in exercise.
COLD with RHF: the right atrial pressure rises disproportionately whereas the increase of stroke volume and CO are almost absolutely the same as in the preceding subgroup. The same is true for OD.
CRLD without RHF: again, insignificant change of right atrial pressure (in fact, this pressure slightly decreased) with marked rise of stroke volume, CO and OD.

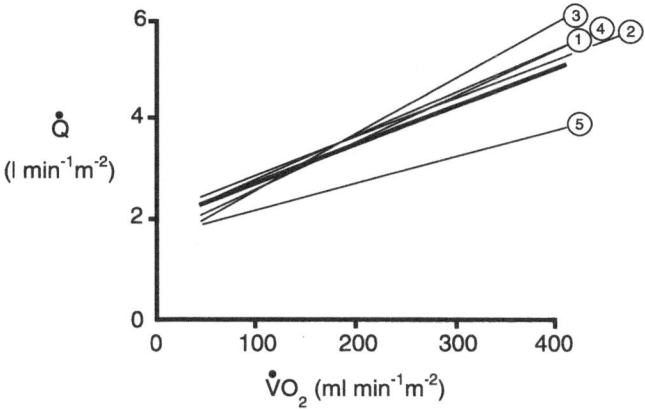

Fig. 1. Relation between oxygen consumption ($\dot{V}O_2$) and cardiac output ($\dot{Q}$) in examined groups of patients. Thick solid line represents this relation in healthy subjects.[17] Thin lines represent this relation in individual subgroups:
1 = compensated patients with COLD;
2 = decompensated patients with COLD;
3 = compensated patients with CRLD;
4 = decompensated patients with CRLD;
5 = cardiac patients.
The last regression line differs significantly from the others.

CRLD with RHF: a marked rise of right atrial pressure but again a proportional increase of cardiac output, CO and OD.

Cardiac patients: the rise of right atrial pressure is similar to that observed in decompensated COLD and CRLD. In contrast to patients with chronic lung diseases, the cardiac patients do not increase their stroke volume at all and the rise of CO and OD is limited.

Briefly summarized, the adaptation of both pulmonary subgroups to the low-level supine exercise is very similar. The differences between COLD and CRLD in absolute values are probably due to the influence of different negative intrathoracic pressures (not measured in our study) and to the fact that the work load of 40 Watts prevailed in COLD whereas 20 Watts were more frequent in CRLD.

The patients with clinical signs of RHF differed from the compensated ones only by an abnormal increase of right atrial pressure. It is to be noted however that preserved blood flow and oxygen delivery is achieved only at the cost of more marked increase of right ventricular work (Fig. 2). Cardiac patients differ from the others by the incapacity to increase adequately the blood flow.

2. Preterminal respiratory and haemodynamic values and their development
The results are summarized in Tables III and IV.
There is only one marked difference between both "pulmonary" subgroups:

Table III: Respiratory and haemodynamic values in three subgroups of patients registered before death.

Value	COLD (16)	CRLD (12)	Cardiac patients (16)	Differences		
				COLD-CRLD	COLD-Cardiac	CRLD-Cardiac
$\overline{P}_{ra}$ (mmHg)	5.70± 5.60	6.10±4.90	11.40±4.60	NS	p<0.01	p<0.05
$\overline{P}_{pa}$ (mmHg)	35.00±14.00	50.00±13.00	48.00±17.00	p<0.05	p<0.05	NS
$\overline{P}_{w}$ (mmHg)	8.90±5.00	13.30± 6.90	30.60±9.50	NS	p<0.001	p<0.001
$\overset{\bullet}{V}O_2$ (ml min^{-1} m^{-2})	142.00±18.00	143.00±30.00	137.00±28.00	NS	NS	NS
PaO_2 (mmHg)	57.00±8.00	62.00±16.00	71.00±8.00	NS	p<0.01	p<0.05
SaO_2 (%)	88.00± 5.00	89.00± 6.00	94.00±2.00	NS	p<0.01	p<0.05
SvO_2 (%)	61.00±7.00	63.00± 4.00	59.00±11.00	NS	NS	NS
$C_{a-v}O_2$ (ml l^{-1})	51.00±11.00	60.50± 8.00	68.60±19.70	NS	p<0.01	NS
Hb (g l^{-1})	144.00±20.00	174.00±33.00	142.00±12.00	p<0.01	NS	p<0.01
$\overset{\bullet}{Q}$ (l min^{-1} m^{-2})	2.97±0.72	2.32± 0.28	2.12±0.51	p<0.05	p<0.01	NS
HR (min^{-1})	94.00±18.00	97.00±13.00	86.00±15.00	NS	NS	NS
SV (ml m^{-2})	33.00±10.00	25.00± 5.00	25.00±9.00	p<0.05	p<0.05	NS
W_R (W m^{-2})	0.19±0.07	0.23± 0.05	0.17±0.07	NS	NS	NS
OD (ml min^{-1} m^{-2})	512.00±117.00	466.00±62.00	386.00±95.00	NS	p<0.01	p<0.05
ODI	3.59± 0.89	3.14±0.34	2.83±0.61	NS	p<0.01	p<0.05

SvO_2 = oxygen saturation of mixed venous blood;

$C_{a-v}O_2$ = arterial oxygen content;

Hb = haemoglobin concentration;

NS = nonsignificant difference.

Remaining abbreviations are the same as in Tables I and II

patients with CRLD have significantly depressed CO and stroke volume whereas these values are normal in COLD. A nearly normal OD in CRLD could be explained by more marked polycythemia and, consequently, higher oxygen concentration. On the other hand, there are numerous differences between these two subgroups and cardiac patients: the latter have higher right atrial pressure, higher arterial oxygen (but some are frankly hypoxaemic in this stage of the disease), they exhibit further slight lowering of CO and in particular of OD. As for the haemodynamic development, there are some elements common for all subgroups:

- a rise of pulmonary arterial hypertension;

Table IV. Respiratory and haemodynamic evolution before preterminal catheterization

Value	COLD (12)		CRLD (9)		Cardiac patients (9)	
	I	II	I	II	I	II
$\overline{P}_{ra}$ (mmHg)	4.10±4.90	5.00±4.90	4.60±3.20	6.80±5.30	5.40±4.50	12.30±5.70^{xxx}
$\overline{P}_{pa}$ (mmHg)	31.00±11.00	36.00±12.00^x	37.00±7.00	52.00±12.00^{xx}	41.00±13.00	50.00±19.00^x
$\overline{P}_{w}$ (mmHg)	7.00±3.00	10.00± 5.00	8.00±4.00	13.00±7.00	24.00± 5.00	32.00±10.00^x
$\dot{V}O_2$ (ml min^{-1} m^{-2})	156.00±29.00	139.00±16.00	158.00±17.00	148.00±30.00	152.00±14.00	139.00±26.00
PaO$_2$ (mmHg)	58.00±7.00	55.00±7.00	67.00±12.00	61.00±13.00	78.00±5.00	71.00±10.00
SaO$_2$ (%)	88.00±5.00	87.00±4.00	92.00±4.00	89.00±5.00^x	95.00± 1.00	94.00±3.00
SvO$_2$ (%)	66.00±5.00	61.00±7.00	68.00±2.00	62.00±4.00	62.00±9.00	53.00±15.00
$C_{a\text{-}v}O_2$ (ml l^{-1})	45.80±11.30	51.50±12.60	53.00±8.20	63.00±7.40^x	64.90±14.40	75.20±22.40^x
Hb (g l^{-1})	154.00±23.00	147.00±21.00	162.00±18.00	182.00±33.00^x	145.00±11.00	142.00±9.00
$\dot{Q}$ (l min^{-1} m^{-2})	3.81±1.09	3.01±0.78^{xx}	2.85±0.44	2.25±0.27^{xx}	2.36± 0.47	1.88±0.42^{xx}
HR (min^{-1})	93.00±14.00	97.00±19.00	86.00±11.00	101.00±13.00^x	89.00±14.00	86.00±12.00
SV (ml m^{-2})	41.00±12.00	32.00±11.00^{xx}	34.00±7.00	23.00±4.00^{xx}	27.00±7.00	22.00±5.00^{xx}
W_r (W m^{-2})	0.22±0.08	0.20±0.06	0.21±0.04	0.23±0.05	0.19±0.08	0.16±0.07
OD (ml min^{-1} m^{-2})	698.00±216.00	524.00±117.00^x	563.00±65.00	466.00±66.00^{xxx}	461.00±106.00	352.00±95.00^{xxx}
ODI	4.33±1.09	3.66±0.97	3.79±0.49	3.39±0.37^x	3.12±0.57	2.67±0.70^x

I = the first catheterization during the course of the disease;
II= preterminal catheterization;
x = p<0.05;
xx = p<0.01;
xxx = p<0.001.
Remaining abbreviations are the same as in the preceding Tables

- slight and insignificant progression of hypoxaemia;
- stepwise decrease of CO and stroke volume;
- drop of OD and ODI;
- the right ventricular work is elevated but there is no further preterminal increase.

Some particular features are however different between the subgroups:

- CO despite its preterminal drop remains within normal limits in COLD but it becomes depressed in CRLD and the cardiacs;
- the right atrial pressure rises significantly only in cardiac patients.
  A brief summary: haemodynamic deterioration occurs in all patients; it is

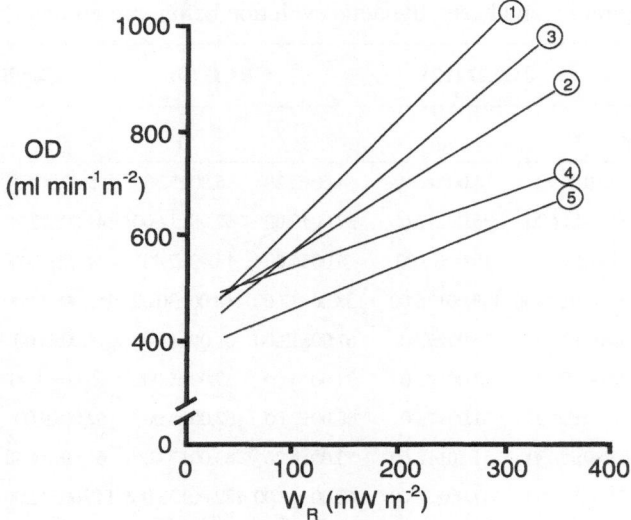

Fig. 2. Relation between right ventricular systolic work (W_R) and oxygen tissue delivery (OD) in examined groups of patients. The numbers refer to the same subgroups as in Fig. 1.

characterized particularly by the decrease of CO and OD. All patient categories however preserve their characteristic haemodynamic features.

Discussion

We have mentioned in the introduction the different opinions concerning the development of pulmonary haemodynamics in COLD which are often controversial. It seems probable that the haemodynamics in not very advanced cases of COLD always free from clinical signs of right heart failure could be stabilized over many years.[36-41] Acute respiratory insufficiency and the recovery from it can change substantially the haemodynamic values[36,37] but the development of the signs of chronic cardiorespiratory failure need not necessarily change haemodynamics. We have found according to other reports that the response of always compensated patients to exercise is entirely normal. Also subjects with clinical signs of RHF are able to develop an adequate blood flow and OD under exercise; this rise is in some cases even higher than normal.

These data concern only the patients with COLD. The situation in other chronic lung diseases has been studied less frequently.

CO in patients with chronic lung fibrosis - both idiopathic and secondary - is also normal on the average.[42-49] It increases also proportionally to the rise of oxygen consumption in exercise[44-47] which corresponds to our results.

It concerns also the subgroup with signs of RHF. However, in most advanced stages of the disease the CO is mostly under normal limits as well as the stroke volume and OD.

CO in chronic thromboembolic disease has seldom been studied. It is normal or even elevated in acute embolism provided that there is no development of RHF[50,52-55] but it seems probable that a tendency to stepwise decrease of CO prevails in chronic cases with pronounced PH.[50,51,53]

The haemodynamic data in so-called primary pulmonary hypertension are sometimes difficult to assess because of the spontaneous variability of haemodynamic values which are more pronounced than in other lung disease.[56-59]

Nevertheless, the tendency to lowered CO in most advanced stages of the disease seems to be proved as does a negative prognostic significance of low CO and stroke volume.[60-62]

A picture of general haemodynamic deterioration is probably common for all chronic lung disease: the deterioration of hypoxaemia, the rise of pulmonary hypertension and the drop of CO, stroke volume and OD were significant in all subgroups. It seems however that COLD represents an exception as regards haemodynamics. COLD exhibits also a preterminal deterioration but both CO and OD remain within normal limits.

Many Authors discussed the "purpose" and mechanism of preserved CO in COLD. The "purpose" is rather clear: normal or slightly increased CO could maintain normal OD despite developing hypoxaemia[63] and this could be regarded as one of the most important compensatory mechanisms. It is usually attributed to hypoxaemia but the direct evidence is lacking. In fact, acute hypoxaemia induces a slight rise of CO[11,13,64,65] whereas acute O_2 inhalation has a depressant effect.[18,65-68] Further, CO can be abnormally high during acute severe hypoxaemia and respiratory insufficiency and it returns to normal level during recovery.[69]

It concerns nevertheless only acute experiments and the clinical situation and its valve in chronic stable hypoxaemia has not been proved. Many authors tried to find a correlation between CO and arterial oxygen saturation but most findings were negative. Moreover, the degree of hypoxaemia is almost the same in COLD and CRLD but the terminal haemodynamics seem to be at least partly different. Therefore, the detailed mechanism of unusual haemodynamic behaviour in decompensated COLD remains relatively obscure.

Decompensated patients both with COLD and CRLD differ from the compensated ones particularly by an abnormal rise of RV filling pressure in exercise. Let us try to interpret this finding.

Normal subjects increase their right ventricular ejection fraction (RVEF) in exercise.[70-74] In other words, they are able to increase the CO in exercise both by tachycardia and by increased stroke output due to enhanced contractility secondary to increased sympathetic tone.

On the other hand, patients with advanced COLD and RV failure are not able to increase their RVEF.[70,72,75] Provided that exertional tachycardia is comparable in compensated and decompensated COLD patients (Table II), the patients with RVF should maintain an adequate stroke output by another manner.

The Frank-Starling law indicates that it is possible only by increasing end-diastolic fibre length, i.e. by increasing the end-diastolic pressure and volume. It is understood that this mechanism requires more energy (see augmented RV stroke work in these patients) but it is effective.

Another mechanism which could contribute to elevated RV end-diastolic pressure in exercise is the RV hypertrophy which could modify the diastolic RV properties.[29]

Our results demonstrate that the regulation of CO in chronic lung diseases is complex; its study could contribute to better understanding of different stages of the disease.

References

1. Richards D.W.: Cardiac output by the catheterization technique in various clinical conditions. Fed. Proc. 1945; 4:215-220
2. McMichael J.: Circulatory failure. Schweiz. Med. Wschr. 1946; 76:851-857
3. Denolin H., De Coster A., Bernard R.: Les causes de l'insuffisance ventriculaire droite dans les pneumopathies chroniques. Prog. Resp. Res. 1971; 6:147-161
4. Fowler N.O., Westcott R.N., Scott R.C., Hess E.: The cardiac output in chronic cor pulmonale. Circulation 1952; 6:888-893
5. Sadoul P., Schrijen F., Uffholz H., Pham Q.T.: Evolution clinique de 195 pulmonaires chroniques soumis à un cathétérisme du coeur droit entre 1957 et 1965. Bull. Physiopath. Resp. 1968; 4:225-238
6. Segel N., Bishop J.M.: The circulation in patients with chronic bronchitis and emphysema at rest and during exercise, with special reference to the influence of changes in blood viscosity and blood volume on the pulmonary circulation. J. Clin. Invest. 1966; 45:1555-1568
7. Harris P., Heath D.: *The human pulmonary circulation*. Edinburgh, Livingstone, 1977; 522-546
8. Herles F., Jezek V., Daum S.: Site of pulmonary resistance in cor pulmonale in chronic bronchitis. Br. Heart J. 1968; 30:654-660
9. Whitaker W.: Pulmonary hypertension in congestive heart failure complicating chronic lung disease. Quart. J. Med. 1954; 23:57-72
10. Lockhart A.: Hémodynamique pulmonaire dans la bronchite chronique. Bull. Physiopath. Resp. 1973; 9:1069-1099
11. Abraham A.S., Hedworth-Whitty R.B., Bishop J.M.: Effects of acute hypoxia and hypervolaemia singly and together, upon the pulmonary circulation in patients with chronic bronchitis. Clin. Sci. 1967; 33:371-380
12. Lockhart A., Tzareva M., Nader F., Leblanc P., Schrijen F., Sadoul P.: Elevated pulmonary artery wedge pressure at rest and during exercise in chronic bronchitis: fact or fancy. Clin. Sci. 1969; 37:503-517
13. Williams J.F., Behnke R.H.: The effect of pulmonary emphysema upon cardiopulmonary hemodynamics at rest and during exercise. Ann. Int. Med. 1964; 60:824-842
14. Harvey R.M., Smith W.M., Parker J.O., Ferrer I.M.: The response of the abnormal heart to

exercise. Circulation 1962; 26:341-362

15. Ferrer I.M., Conroy R.J., Harvey R.M.: Some effects of digoxin upon the heart and circulation in man. Digoxin in combined (left and right) ventricular failure. Circulation 1960; 21:372-385

16. Degré S., Sergysels R., Messin R., et al.: Hemodynamic responses to physical training in patients with chronic lung disease. Am. Rev. Resp. Dis. 1974; 110:395-402

17. Lockhart A.: Facteurs limitant l'exercice dans les bronchopneumopathies obstructives chroniques. Bull. Eur. Physiopath. Resp. 1979; 15:305-317

18. Horsfield K., Segel N., Bishop J.M.: The pulmonary circulation in chronic bronchitis at rest and during exercise breathing air and 80% oxygen. Clin. Sci. 1968; 34:473-483

19. Light R.W., Mintz H.M., Linden G.S., Brown S.E.: Hemodynamics of patients with severe chronic obstructive pulmonary disease during progressive upright exercise. Am. Rev. Resp. Dis. 1984; 130:391-395

20. Weitzenblum E., El Gharbic T., Vanderenne A., Blegar A., Hirth C., Oudet P.: Pulmonary haemodynamic changes during muscular exercise in non-decompensated chronic bronchitis. Bull. Physiopath. Resp. 1972; 8:49-71

21. Perrin-Fayolle M., Kofman J., Cassan G., Brun J.: Dépistage par l'épreuve d'effort des stades initiaux de l'hypertension pulmonaire au cours de la bronchite chronique. Prog. Resp. Res. 1971; 6:255-270

22. Burrows B., Kettel L.J., Niden A.H., Rabinowitz M., Diener C.F.: Patterns of cardiovascular dysfunction in chronic obstructive lung disease. New Engl. J. Med. 1972; 286:912-918

23. Filley G.F., Beckwitt H.J., Reeves J.T., Mitchells R.S.: Chronic obstructive bronchopulmonary disease. II. Oxygen transport in two clinical types. Am. J. Med. 1968; 44:26-38

24. Howard P.: Aetiological factors in hypoxic cor pulmonale. Prog. Resp. Res. 1985; 20:49-54

25. Schrijen F., Henriquez A., Poincelot F., Polu J.M.: Hemodynamic evaluation in patients with chronic lung disease. Prog. Resp. Res. 1985; 20:144-149

26. Weitzenblum E., Sautegeau A., Ehrhart M., Mammosser M.: Long-term course of pulmonary hemodynamics in chronic obstructive pulmonary disease. Prog. Resp. Res. 1985; 20:150-156

27. Finlay M., Middleton H.C., Peake M.D., Howard P.: Cardiac output, pulmonary hypertension, hypoxaemia and survival in patients with chronic obstructive airways disease. Eur. J. Resp. Dis. 1983; 64:252-263

28. Jezek V., Schrijen F., Sadoul P.: Action hemodynamique du pindolol chez des broncho-pneumopathies chroniques. Bull. Physiopath. Resp. 1972; 8:111-126

29. Jezek V., Schrijen F., Sadoul P.: Right ventricular function and pulmonary hemodynamics during exercise in patients with chronic obstructive bronchopulmonary disease. Cardiology 1973; 58:20-31

30. Jezek V., Schrijen F.: Haemodynamic effect of deslanoside at rest and during exercise in patients with chronic bronchitis. Br. Heart J. 1973; 35:2-8

31. Jezek V., Schrijen F.: Left ventricular function in chronic obstructive pulmonary disease with and without cardiac failure. Clin. Sci. Molec. Med. 1973; 45:267-279

32. Yang S.S., Bentivoglio L.G., Maranhao V., Goldberg H.: *From cardiac catheterization data to haemodynamic parameters*. Philadelphia, Davis 1972; 1-307

33. Wallenstein S., Zucker C.L., Fleiss J.L.: Some statistical methods useful in circulation research. Circulation Res. 1980; 47:1-9

34. Remington R.D., Schork M.A.: *Statistics with applications to the biological and health sciences*. New York, Prentice-Hall 1985

35. Ekelund L.G., Holmgren A.: Central hemodynamics during exercise. Circulation Res. 1967; (Suppl) 20-21:33-43

36. Jezek V., Ourednik A.: Development of pulmonary hypertension in chronic cor pulmonale and

emphysema; its relationship to the development of chronic respiratory insufficiency. Bull. Physiopath. Resp. 1968; 4:297-305

37. Weitzenblum E., Jezek V.: Evolution of pulmonary hypertension in chronic respiratory diseases. Bull. Eur. Physiopath. Resp. 1984; 20:73-81

38. Schrijen F., Henriquez A., Poincelot F., Polu J.M.: Hemodynamic evolution in patients with chronic lung disease. Prog. Resp. Res. 1985; 20:144-149

39. Weitzenblum E., Loiseau A., Hirth C., Mirhom R., Rasaholinjanahary J.: Course of pulmonary hemodynamics in patients with chronic obstructive pulmonary disease. Chest 1979; 75:656-662

40. Schrijen F., Uffholtz H., Polu J.M., Poincelot F.: Pulmonary and systemic hemodynamic evolution in chronic bronchitis. Am. Rev. Resp. Dis. 1978; 117:25-31

41. Weitzenblum E., Sautegeau A., Ehrhart M., Mammosser M.: Long-term course of pulmonary hemodynamics in chronic obstructive pulmonary disease. Prog. Resp. Res. 1985; 20:150-156

42. Jezek V., Fucik J., Michaljanic A., Jezkova L.: The prognostic significance of functional tests in kryptogenic fibrosing alveolitis. Bull. Eur. Physiopath. Resp. 1980; 16:711-720

43. Jezek V.: The prognosis and development of pulmonary hypertension in idiopathic diffuse interstitial lung fibrosis. G. Ital. Cardiol. 1984; 14 (Suppl) 1:39-45

44. Hawrylkiewicz I., Izdebska-Makosa Z., Brebska E., Zielinski J.: Pulmonary haemodynamics at rest and on exercise in patients with idiopathic pulmonary fibrosis. Bull. Eur. Physiopath. Resp. 1982; 18:403-410

45. Weitzenblum E., Ehrhart M., Rasaholnjanahary J., Hirth C.: Pulmonary hemodynamics in idiopathic pulmonary fibrosis and other interstitial pulmonary diseases. Respiration 1983; 44:118-127

46. Widimsky J., Riedel M., Stanek V.: Central haemodynamics during exercise in patients with restrictive pulmonary disease. Bull. Eur. Physiopath. Resp. 1977; 13:369-379

47. Gimenez M., Uffholtz H., Schrijen F.: Résponses ventilatoires et cardio-respiratoires des restrictifs à l'exercice musculaire. Bull. Eur. Physiopath. Resp. 1977; 13:355-367

48. De Coster A., Denolin H., Rutsaert J., Derriks R.: Répercussions hémodynamiques des fibroses interstitielles diffuses. Poumon 1965; 21:601-618

49. Daum S., Sperber H., Goerg R., Schlehe H., Harlacher A., Steuer G.: Präkäpilläre pulmonale hypertension bei chronischen idiopathischen fibrosierenden Alveolitiden ohne und mit Wabenlunge. In: S. Daum (Ed.) *Präkäpilläre pulmonale Hypertonie*, München, Dustri 1977; 103-119

50. Tartulier M., Boutarin J., Ritz B.: Chronic pulmonary thromboembolism. G. Ital. Cardiol. 1984; 14: Suppl. 1, 13-21

51. Riedel M., Stanek V., Widimsky J., Prerovsky I.: Long-term follow-up of patients with pulmonary thromboembolism. Chest 1982; 81:151-158

52. Widimsky J.: Mechanisms in embolic pulmonary hypertension. In: C.A. Wagenvoort and H.Denolin, (Ed.) *Pulmonary Circulation advances and controversies*. Amsterdam, Elsevier, 1989; 75-86

53. McIntyre K.M., Sasahara A.A.: The hemodynamic response to pulmonary embolism in patients without prior cardiopulmonary disease. Am. J. Cardiol. 1971; 28:288-294

54. McIntyre K.M., Sasahara A.A.: Haemodynamics and ventricular responses to pulmonary embolism. Prog. Cardiovasc. Dis. 1974; 3:175-190

55. Stanek V., Riedel M., Widimsky J.: Haemodynamic monitoring in acute pulmonary embolism. Bull. Eur. Physiopath. Resp. 1978; 14:561-572

56. Rich S., Martinez J., Lam W., Rosen K.M.: Captopril as treatment for patients with pulmonary hypertension. Problem of variability in assessing chronic drug treatment. Br. Heart J. 1982; 48:272-277

57. Rich S., D'Alonzo G.E., Dantzker D.R., Levy P.S.: Magnitude and implications of spontaneous haemodynamic variability in primary pulmonary hypertension. Am. J. Cardiol. 1985; 55:159-163

58. Jezkova J., Michaljanic A., Jezek V.: Natural variability of pulmonary haemodynamics (Abstract). Eur. Heart J. 1987; 8, (suppl.2), 40

59. Schrjjen F., Jezkova J.: Natural variability of pulmonary haemodynamics. Eur. Heart J. 1988; 9 (Suppl. J).19-22

60. Rich S., Brundage B.H.: The pharmacological treatment of primary pulmonary hypertension. In: Begofsky E.H., (Ed.) *Abnormal pulmonary circulation*, New York, Livingstone, 1986; 283-311

61. Rich S., Levy P.S.: Characteristics of surviving and nonsurviving patients with pulmonary hypertension. Am. J. Med. 1984; 76:573-578

62. Kanemoto N., Sasamoto H.: Pulmonary hemodynamics in primary pulmonary hypertension. Jpn. Heart J. 1979; 20:395-405

63. Bergofsky E.H.: Tissue oxygen delivery and cor pulmonale in chronic obstructive pulmonary disease. New Engl. J. Med. 1983; 308:1092-1094

64. Westcott R.N., Fowler N.O., Scott R.C., Hauenstein V.D., McGuire J.: Anoxia and human pulmonary vascular resistance. J. Clin. Invest. 1951; 30:957-970

65. Fishman A.P., Fritts H.W., Cournand A.: Effects of acute hypoxia on the pulmonary circulation. Circulation 1960; 22:204-215

66. Cotes J.E., Pisa Z., Thomas A.J.: Effect of breathing oxygen upon cardiac output, heart rate, ventilation, systemic and pulmonary blood pressure in patients with chronic lung disease. Clin. Sci. 1963; 25:305-321

67. Kitchen A.H., Lowther C.P., Matthews M.B.: The effects of exercise and of breathing oxygen-enriched air on the pulmonary circulation in emphysema. Clin. Sci. 1961; 21:93-106

68. Timms R.M., Khaja F.U., Williams G.W., and the Nocturnal Oxygen Therapy Trial Group: Hemodynamic response to oxygen therapy in chronic obstructive pulmonary disease. Ann. Intern. Med. 1985; 102:29-36

69. Lockhart A., Tzareva M., Schrijen F., Sadoul P.: Etudes hémodynamiques des décompensations respiratoires aiguës des bronchopneumopathies chroniques. Bull. Physiopath. Resp. 1967; 3:645-667

70. Olvey S.K., Reduto L.A., Stevens P.M., Deaton W.J., Miller R.R.: First pass radionuclide assessment of right and left ventricular ejection fraction in chronic pulmonary disease. Chest 1980; 78:4-9

71. Maddahi J., Berman D.S., Matsuoka D.T., Waxman A.D., Forrester J.S., Swan H.J.C.: Right ventricular ejection fraction during exercise in normal subjects and in coronary artery disease patients: assessment by multiple-gated equilibrium scintigraphy. Circulation 1980; 62:133-140

72. Slutsky R., Hooper W., Ackerman W., Moser K.: The response of right ventricular size, function, and pressure to supine exercise: A comparison of patients with chronic obstructive lung disease and normal subjects. Eur. J. Nucl. Med. 1982; 7:553-558

73. Morrison D., Sorensen S., Caldwell J., Wright A.L., Ritchie J., Kennedy J.W., Hamilton G.: The normal right ventricular response to supine exercise. Chest 1982; 82:686-691

74. Morise A.P., Goodwin C.: Exercise radionuclide angiography in patients with mitral stenosis: value of right ventricular response. Am. Heart J. 1986; 112:509-517

75. Morrison D.A., Adcock K., Collins C.M., Goldman S., Caldwell J.H., Schwarz M.I.: Right ventricular dysfunction and the exercise limitation of chronic obstructive pulmonary disease. J. Am. Coll. Cardiol. 1987; 9:1219-1229

10. Right Ventricular Function in Chronic Obstructive Pulmonary Disease

W. MacNee, K. Skwarski

Department of Respiratory Medicine, City Hospital, Edinburgh, UK

Supported by Norman Salvesen Emphysema Fund and the British Heart Foundation

Introduction

Chronic obstructive pulmonary disease (COPD), resulting largely from chronic bronchitis and emphysema, is a common condition in Scotland, accounting for 465 deaths/100,000 of the population.[1]

In some patients progression of the condition leads to chronic hypoxaemia, with or without hypercapnia. Once respiratory failure has developed, such patients are at risk of developing "cor pulmonale" or "pulmonary heart disease", terms which have been much misused in the literature. To some physicians these terms indicate a patient with chronic lung disease who has peripheral oedema, raised jugular venous pressure, with or without clinical signs of right ventricular hypertrophy or pulmonary hypertension. To others they suggest the presence of pulmonary hypertension in a patient with COPD.

Few use the term "cor pulmonale" according to the WHO definition which is *right ventricular hypertrophy resulting from disorders that affect either the structure or the function on the lungs.*[2] This latter pathological definition is rarely clinically useful and should perhaps be abandoned in favour of a statement of the facts in each individual case, eg. a patient with COPD and pulmonary hypertension, or clinical signs of right ventricular hypertrophy. However, it would be difficult to forsake the term "cor pulmonale" entirely, since it has become entrenched in the literature. Perhaps its use could be confined to the clinical syndrome of cardiomegaly, raised jugular venous pressure and oedema in a patient with chronic lung disease and respiratory failure.

The classical view of the development of "cor pulmonale" is that hypoxaemia results in pulmonary vaso-constriction, leading to pulmonary hypertension, at first on exercise and later at rest[3] as structural changes develop in the intima which narrow the small pulmonary vessels.[4]

It has been proposed that the consequence of this increased pressure load is the development of right ventricular hypertrophy and eventually clinical signs of right ventricular failure, often occurring during an exacerbation of COPD. However, whether the clinical syndrome of "cor pulmonale" represents true right ventricular failure, remains controversial.[5,6] Whatever the pathogenesis of the oedema in patients with COPD, its presence results in a high mortality, only 45% of such patients surviving for 2 years, compared with a 69% survival at 2 years in patients without oedema.[7] The presence of pulmonary arterial hypertension in patients with COPD also worsens survival.[8]

Clearly a greater understanding of the clinical syndrome of "cor pulmonale", in particular whether this develops primarily as a result right heart failure may lead to more rational therapy for this condition.

Previous Studies of Right Ventricular Function

Assessment of right ventricular performance remains a problem, principally due to the variable and irregular shape of the chamber even in health[9], making measurements of chamber volume difficult by contrast angiography.[10] In general, the thin-walled right ventricle which contracts against the low pressure pulmonary circulation, is considered to be more compliant than the thicker-walled left ventricle. The right ventricular geometric configuration is therefore thought to be more suited to ejecting large volumes of blood, with minimal myocardial shortening, and therefore can adapt to considerable variations in the systemic venous return, without producing large changes in filling pressures.[11,12] However, it is less able to cope with high afterload pressures.[12,13]

In the dog active constriction of the pulmonary artery, producing even small changes in the pulmonary arterial pressure, results in a rapid decrease in stroke volume (Fig. 1), whereas the left ventricle maintains its stroke volume relatively well, despite increases in systemic pressure. By contrast increasing ventricular pre-load or filling pressure by fourfold, as a result of volume expansion, produces an increase in left ventricular work, which is five times that of the right ventricle.[14]

It seems reasonable therefore to assume that a chronic increase in pressure load will lead to changes in the configuration, mass and function of the right ventricle. However, the pulmonary arterial pressure in most patients with COPD and respiratory failure is not markedly elevated,[15] and the rate of progression of pulmonary arterial hypertension in such patients is slow. Weitzenblum et al.[16] studied the change in pulmonary haemodynamics in patients with COPD over an average of 5 years, and found that the pulmonary arterial pressure increased by a mean of only 3 mmHg/year. However, the mean increase in pressure was >5mmHg

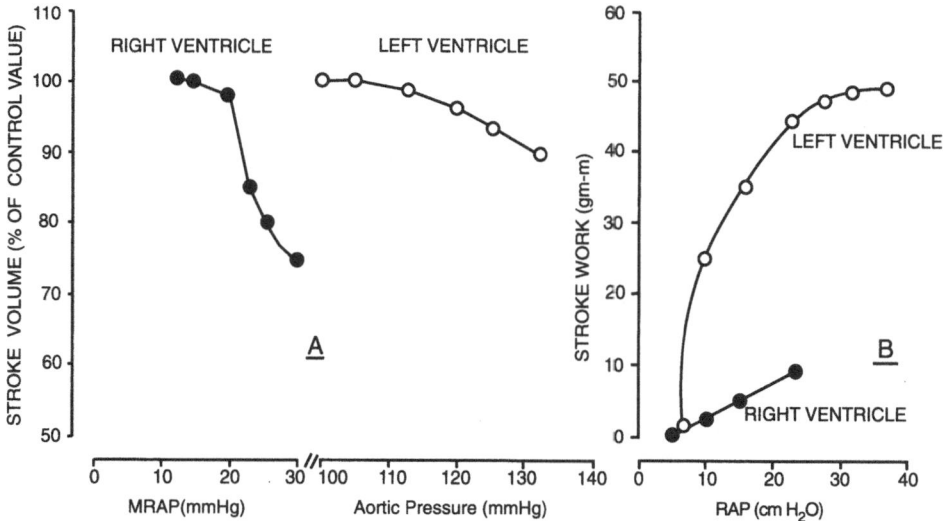

Fig. 1. The effects of increasing afterload (A) and pre-load (B) on the right and left ventricles in the dog. Stroke volume decreases rapidly when afterload is increased in the right ventricle, in contrast to the left ventricle, which maintains stroke volume reasonably well against an augmented afterload (A). In contrast, the stroke work of the left ventricle increases dramatically when pre-load is increased, which is not the case with the right ventricle (B) (after McFadden ER and Braunwald E.).[14]

in only 33% of these patients. By contrast, Schrijen et al[17] found no significant deterioration in pulmonary haemodynamics in a group of patients with COPD studied over 3 years, even in those with pulmonary hypertension. Thus the effect on right ventricular function of the moderate pulmonary hypertension which is slowly progressive in patients with COPD, is likely to be different from the effects of acute pulmonary hypertension, which occurs in massive pulmonary embolism[18], or the effect of the systemic levels of pulmonary arterial pressure which occur chronically in primary pulmonary hypertension.[19]

Pulmonary Haemodynamics in COPD

Patients with mild COPD, without severe hypoxaemia or hypercapnia have a normal or low cardiac output.[20-26]

Right atrial and right ventricular end-diastolic pressures are normal, and pulmonary arterial pressure is only slightly elevated, but is inappropriately high for the level of the cardiac output. Pulmonary vascular resistance is therefore normal or only slightly elevated when measured at rest in such patients. During exercise the pulmonary arterial pressure rises to abnormal levels. However, as in normal subjects, the increase in cardiac output is normal relative to the increase in oxygen consumption.[25-26] Right ventricular end-diastolic pressure and right ventricular stroke work, both of which are normal at rest in patients with mild to moderately severe COPD, rise during exercise[25], due to an increase in pressure work against a higher pulmonary arterial pressure.

However, the relationship between the right ventricular end-diastolic pressure and stroke work index suggests that these patients operate on an extension of their normal right ventricular function curve.[25] As airflow limitation and arterial blood gas abnormalities worsen, particularly when chronic hypoxaemia develops, pulmonary hypertension is present at rest, and worsens with exercise.[24-25,27]

However, at rest, right ventricular end-diastolic pressure is normal, even in those patients with clinical evidence of right ventricular hypertrophy, who have had episodes of peripheral oedema in the past.[25] The presence of a normal right ventricular end-diastolic pressure has been presumed to reflect a normal right ventricular end-diastolic volume.[27]

Pulmonary Haemodynamics in Patients with COPD and Oedema

Relatively few haemodynamic studies have been made in patients with COPD who were considered to have "right ventricular failure".[22,28-31] Such patients have a lower arterial oxygen tension and a higher pulmonary arterial pressure and pulmonary vascular resistance at rest than those without evidence of oedema.[31] Further desaturation is usual during exercise, associated with a rise in pulmonary arterial pressure and resistance.[22,25,31]

Right ventricular end-diastolic and right atrial pressures are often elevated; however, the slope of the relationship between the right ventricular stroke work and the ventricular end-diastolic pressure is similar in patients with severe COPD with and without oedema.[25]

Right Ventricular Ejection Fraction in Patients with COPD

Contrast angiography has been used to measure right ventricular volumes. However, the measurement requires certain geometric assumptions which may not be justified because of the irregular right ventricular shape.[9,32] Radionuclide ventriculography avoids this problem to some extent. First pass and gated ventriculography can be used to assess right ventricular performance using [99m]Technetium labelled red blood cells, or human serum albumin (HSA). However, both methods have advantages and disadvantages. The principal disadvantage of the first pass technique, is the difficulty in performing sequential measurements, requiring repeated bolus injections of radiotracers, and an increase in the radiation burden to the patient. Furthermore, the short acquisition time results in low counts and statistical uncertainty in calculating the ejection fraction. However, repeated measurements can be undertaken using an [81m]Krypton infusion, rather than [99m]Technetium labelled HSA or erythrocytes. The principal advantage of the first pass technique is that the ventricles can be separated both in time and in space, avoiding the problems of overlap between the two chambers.

In order to separate the ventricles, using the equilibrium technique, a left anterior oblique view is used. However, corrections must still be made for background counts, and two regions of interest must be drawn at end-systole and end-diastole to avoid overlap of the right atrium and right ventricle.[33,34] The equilibrium technique provides better count statistics, since data from several hundred cardiac cycles are acquired. Moreover, repeated measurements can be made over three hours following a single injection of a radiotracer.When reporting results of measurements of right ventricular ejection fraction (RVEF), measured by radionuclide ventriculography, it is essential to assess the reproducibility of the technique. We have previously reported a good correlation between the RVEF measured by either the first pass or the equilibrium techniques (Fig. 2).[34]

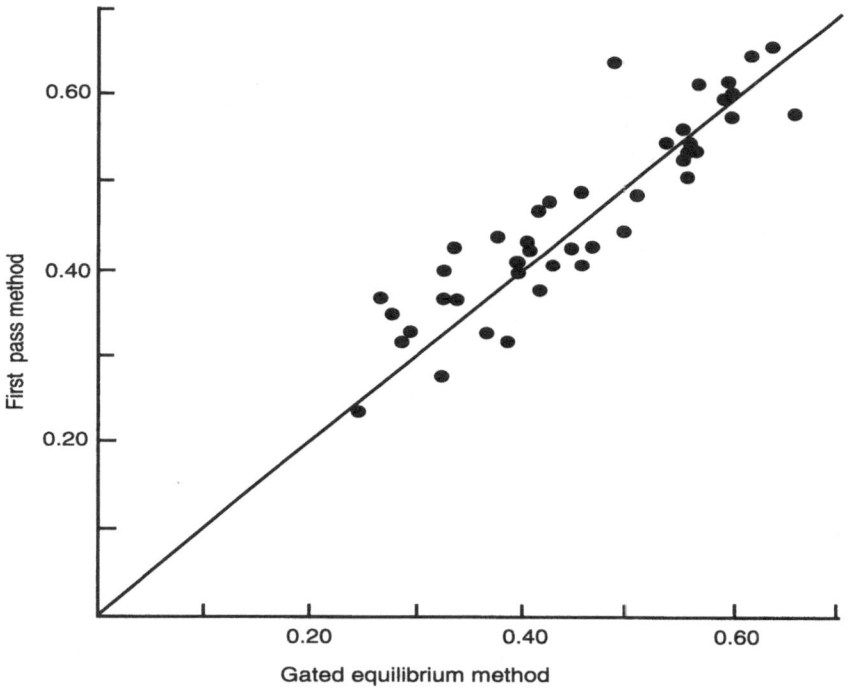

Fig. 2. Comparison of the right ventricular ejection fraction (RVEF) by the first pass and equilibrium methods. The line of identity is shown. The mean difference in RVEF by the two methods was 0.04 (n = 43, r = 0.91, p<0.001).

The intra-observer variability measured in 40 equilibrium studies was 0.03, and the inter-observer variability was 0.04.

Although the reproducibility over time was good when measurements were made on two separate occasions when the patients remained supine, the technique was less reproducible when measured in the same individual on different days[35] which may be due to an inherent variability in RVEF, or reflect positional changes which result in variable ventricular and atrial overlap.

In 30 normal subjects (mean age 39.4±12.5 yrs) with a mean left ventricular ejection fraction (LVEF) of 0.57±0.07 (SD), the mean RVEF was 0.5±0.09 (range 0.47-0.83).[33]

Thus our lower limit of normal for RVEF (2 standard deviations below the mean) is 0.40 when measured at rest. RVEF increased by at least 7% during exercise (RVEF during exercise 0.62± 0.06). In 100 patients with chronic bronchitis and emphysema (Table I), RVEF measured at rest by gated equilibrium radionuclide ventriculography, was 0.44±0.01.

Although this value was significantly lower than in normal subjects ($p<0.01$), only 35 of the 100 patients had a low RVEF and there was significant correlation between RVEF and the arterial oxygen tension in the patients with COPD ($r = 0.41$; $p<0.001$). When these 100 patients were divided on the basis of the presence or absence of oedema indicating "cor pulmonale", most of those with oedema ($n = 28$) had a low RVEF. During exercise the majority of patients with COPD do not show the normal increase in either RVEF or LVEF (Fig. 3).

In a group of 25 patients with COPD, only 7 had a normal response to exercise. Interestingly, the change in arterial oxygen saturation correlated with the change in RVEF ($r = 0.50$; $p<0.02$).

The quoted values of RVEF in patients with COPD vary in the literature[36-49] (Table II). Few of these patients have values which are as those reported in patients with right ventricular infarcts.[50-51]

Table I. RVEF and LVEF in 100 patients with chronic bronchitis and emphysema

	Mean± SD	Range
Age (yr)	62.00±8.0	41.00-80.00
PaO$_2$ (kPa)	7.30±1.30	4.70-11.30
PaCO$_2$ (kPa)	6.40±1.20	4.40-10.80
FEV$_1$ (l)	0.75±0.38	0.30- 2.90
FVC (l)	1.98±0.80	0.70- 4.70
RVEF	0.44±0.10	0.24- 0.62
LVEF	0.44±0.11	0.24- 0.79

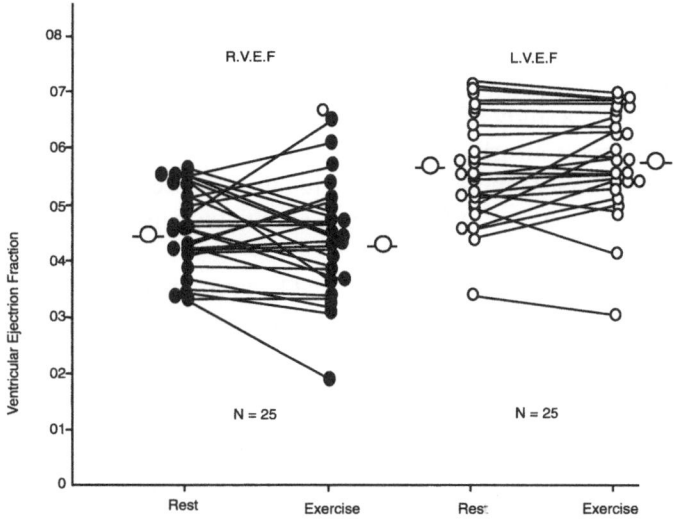

Fig. 3. Right (RVEF) and left (LVEF) ventricular ejection fractions at rest and during supine exercise when breathing air in 25 patients with chronic bronchitis and emphysema. Mean values of RVEF and LVEF (-o-) did not change during exercise, although the response to exercise was very variable.

Table II. The quoted values of RVEF with COPD vary in the literarure.

Authors	No. of patiens	RVEF at rest	RVEF on exercise
Ellis et al.[36]	39	0.47±0.02	-
Olvey et al.[37]	18	0.43±0.02	0.44±0.03
Berger et al.[38]	36	0.47±0.12	-
Matthay et al.[39]	30	0.49±0.01	0.47±0.02
Slutsky et al.[40]	20	0.46±0.09	-
Mather et al.[41]	15	0.34±0.08	-
Houper et al.[42]	14	0.37±0.14	-
Dahlstrom et al.[43]	10	0.43±0.14	-
Erickson et al.[44]	10	0.38±0.11	-
Brown et al.[45]	12	0.41±0.04	-
Tuxen et al.[46]	9	0.33±0.08	-
Brent et al.[47]	30	0.41±0.07	-
Burghuber et al.[48]	24	0.44±0.03	-
Morrison et al.[49]	9	0.54±0.07	-

It seems in most studies that RVEF correlates with the severity of COPD. We found weak correlations between RVEF and the arterial oxygen and carbon dioxide tensions (PaO_2, $PaCO_2$).[52]

Berger et al.[53], in a study of 36 patients with COPD found that those with severe airflow limitation (arbitrarily defined as FEV_1 <1 litre) had a lower RVEF than those whose pulmonary function was less impaired. Moreover, the presence of right ventricular hypertrophy on ECG was also associated with a low RVEF. We were unable to confirm these findings.[52]

The correlation between RVEF and PaO_2, and between the change in right ventricular ejection fraction on exercise and the change in SaO_2 suggests that RVEF relates to the clinical type in patients with COPD.

Indeed, those patients with a normal response to exercise appeared to be of the "pink and puffing" type,[54] whereas those whose RVEF did not rise normally during exercise were of the "blue and bloated" type. However, the presence or absence of emphysema, at least as measured by CT lung density,[55] does not correlate with the RVEF. Nor does the presence of emphysema correlate with the level of the pulmonary arterial pressure, or relate to the clinical type in patients with COPD.[56]

Relationship between RVEF and Pulmonary Arterial Pressure

The right ventricular hypothesis of the development of cor pulmonale,[6] suggests that RVEF is highly after-load dependent. However, data in the literature indicates a wide variation in the correlation between pulmonary arterial pressure and RVEF (Table III).[36,43,48,57-63]

Our own study in 100 patients with COPD showed no significant correlation between simultaneous measurements of RVEF and pulmonary arterial pressure (Fig. 4), although a weak but significant correlation was present between RVEF and the pulmonary vascular resistance.[64]

Although differences between the techniques used to measure RVEF or differences between the patients studied may account for this variation, there may be a more fundamental reason why RVEF should not be expected to correlate with pulmonary arterial pressure.

RVEF depends not only an afterload, but also on the pre-load and on ventricular contractility. Moreover, the pulmonary arterial pressure or the pulmonary vascular resistance are not accurate measurements of the right ventricular afterload, which by definition, is the stress or tension acting on the fibres of the right ventricular wall, immediately after the onset of shortening.[65]

Thus the true right ventricular afterload is the force per unit cross-sectional area acting on the right ventricular wall.[66]

Assessment of right ventricular wall stress requires measurement of both the right ventricular volume and the wall thickness. Thus pulmonary arterial pressure

Table III. Relationship between RVEF and pulmonary arterial pressure.

Author	No. of patients/ subjects	Patient type	Correlation coefficient
Ellis et al.[36]	35	COPD	-0.32 (NS)
Winzelberg et al.[57]	56	VHD	0.23 (NS)
Korr et al.[58]	37	Normal subjects, IHD, VHD	-0.82 (p<0.001)
Friedman et al.[59]	49	Cardiomyopathy, VHD, IHD	-0.56 (p<0.05)
Morrison et al.[49]	39	Cardiomyopathy, VHD, IHD	-0.57 (p<0.05)
Morrison et al.[60]	9	Normal subjects	NS
Dahlstrom et al.[43]	10	Chronic lung disease	-0.75 (p<0.05)
Brent et al.[61]	30	COPD	-0.74 (p<0.01)
Mahler et al.[62]	12	COPD	-0.48 (NS)
Burghuber et al.[63]	14	COPD	-0.75 (p<0.01)
Burghuber et al.[48]	24	COPD	-0.73 (p<0.001)

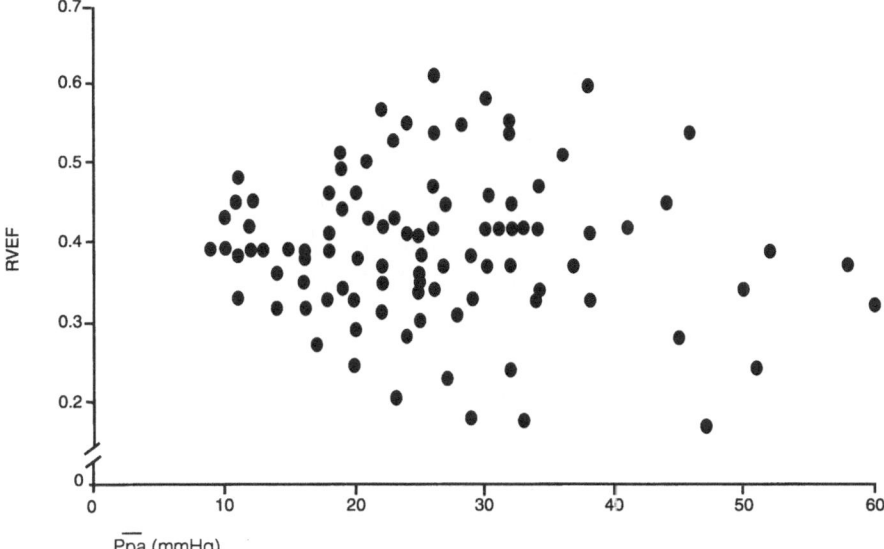

Fig. 4. The relationship between simultaneous measurements of right ventricular ejection fraction (RVEF) and mean pulmonary arterial pressure (Ppa) in 100 patients with chronic obstructive pulmonary disease (r = .0.07, p>0.05).

has been used to estimate right ventricular afterload but represents only a fraction of the true afterload, and assumes that intra-cavitary pressure closely approximates to transmural pressure.[67] Pulmonary vascular resistance may be a slightly more accurate reflection of the true right ventricular afterload, but it is still an approximation.

In a study by Gunter and Grossman, in patients with aortic stenosis and left ventricular pressure overload, left ventricular systolic pressure did not correlate with left ventricular ejection fraction.[68]

However, when the mean mid wall circumferential wall stress, a measure of the true afterload was measured, there was a highly significant correlation between wall stress and left ventricular ejection fraction.[68] Thus RVEF should not be regarded as a non-invasive technique to measure pulmonary arterial pressure.

The Effect of Pulmonary Hypertension on Right Ventricular Function

RVEF is a measure of global right ventricular performance and at least in our studies, does not correlate with the pulmonary arterial pressure. To measure the "contractility" or inotropic state of the right ventricle, as distinct from its performance, it is necessary to measure a function of the right ventricle which is independent of change in pre- or afterload.

Assessing ventricular contractility is difficult in man, even in the left ventricle. However, probably the best measurement is the relationship between the pressure and volume of the ventricle at end-systole.[69] The concept of the end-systolic pressure/volume (PV) relationship, was first developed in isolated heart preparations,[70] but is also applicable in intact man.[71]

The end-systolic P/V relationship in the left ventricle has been shown to be independent of the pre-load and afterload.[72] Thus for a given contractility, the relationship remains linear if afterload is varied, hence the P/V ratio remains constant. Heart failure decreases the slope of the relationship, shifting it to the right, and inotropic drugs shift the relationship to the left, increasing its slope.[73]

Peak systolic pressure can also be substituted for end-systolic pressure without changing the validity of the relationship.[74] Although the slope of the end-systolic P/V relationship is a measure of contractility, this requires assessment of the P/V relationship under different loading conditions, and necessitates infusions of vasodilators.

For this reason the P/V point has been used as an estimate of contractility since clearly a small ventricular volume for a given outflow pressure indicates more complete ventricular emptying, suggesting increased contractility.

Using a combination of measurements of right ventricular systolic pressure and right ventricular volume measurements derived from stroke volume measurements made by Swan-Ganz catheter and radionuclide RVEF, we have been able to calculate the right ventricular end-systolic pressure/volume relationship in patients with COPD and determine the effect of pulmonary hypertension on this relationship. We have shown that infusions of the vasodilator sodium nitroprusside in 10 patients with COPD and pulmonary hypertension reduced the pulmonary arterial pressure from 30±6 to 22±6 mmHg (p<0.01) and the total pulmonary vascular resistance from 540±126 to 400±140 dynes s.cm^{-5} (p<0.001).[75]

Despite a fall in pulmonary vascular resistance, the right ventricular end-systolic pressure/volume ratio did not change following afterload reduction (Fig. 5). Moreover, the slopes of the individual pressure/volume relationships following sodium nitroprusside infusion were above unity in the majority suggesting relatively well preserved right ventricular contractility in these patients.

In a larger group of 20 patients with severe COPD (FEV$_1$ 0.7±0.1 l, PaO$_2$ 7.1±1.1 kPa, PaCO$_2$ 6.6±1.1 kPa) and pulmonary hypertension, who all had a past history of oedema, but were stable when studied, the P/V relationship was to the left of the mean value calculated for normal subjects, in spite of the presence of pulmonary hypertension, suggesting preservation of right ventricular contractility.[64] Although other studies[61] have shown the P/V relationship to be increased in patients with COPD and pulmonary hypertension, suggesting depressed right ventricular con-

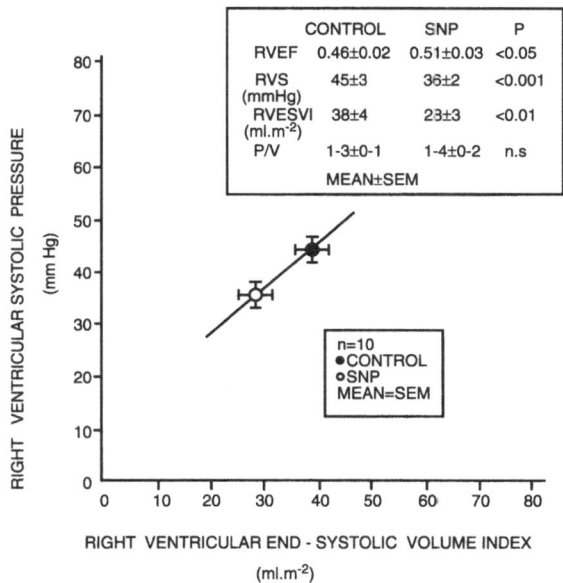

Fig. 5. Sodium nitroprusside (SNP) displaced the mean right ventricular end-systolic pressure/volume point in 10 patients with chronic bronchitis and emphysema downwards and to the left. However, since the right ventricular systolic pressure (RVSP) and right ventricular end-systolic volume index (RV$_{ESVI}$) were both reduced by similar amounts, there was no significant change in the right ventricular end-systolic pressure volume index (P/V).

126

tractility, a more recent study in patients with COPD supports our study by showing a similar P/V relationship in patients with and without pulmonary hypertension.[48] We have also studied the change in the P/V relationship during exercise in 25 patients with COPD. In this study, despite a large increase in the pulmonary arterial pressure during exercise, few patients had a large increase in the right ventricular end-systolic pressure (Fig. 6).[64]

In addition, the slope of the relationship between the right ventricular work index and the end-diastolic pressure in patients with COPD was similar to that in normal subjects, again suggesting normal right ventricular performance, even in the face of an augmented pressure work.[64]

Oxygen (2 l/minute, 1 hour) when given at rest to 8 patients with COPD produced a fall in pulmonary arterial pressure from 30±3 to 25±2 mmHg (p<0.05) and in total pulmonary vascular resistance from 570±67 to 477±51 dynes s.cm[-5]. In spite of these changes the RVEF did not change and the right ventricular end-systolic volume also fell, resulting in no change in the pressure/volume ratio. Thus oxygen acts as mild pulmonary vasodilator in these subjects, but did not change right ventricular contractility.[54,76]

During exercise, oxygen reduced the rise in pulmonary arterial pressure which occurs in patients with COPD and although it prevented the fall in RVEF, which occurred during exercise breathing air in the same patients, it did not normalise the

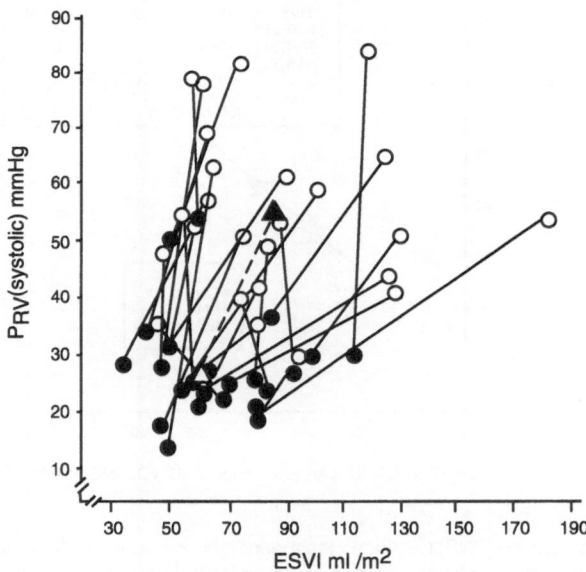

Fig. 6. The right ventricular end-systolic pressure volume relationship at rest (•) and during exercise (o) in 24 patients with chronic obstructive pulmonary disease. The mean values at rest (Δ) and during exercise (▲) are shown.

response of the RVEF to exercise.[54] Thus although we found a relationship between RVEF and PaO_2,[52] the effect on the RVEF when hypoxia was relieved, does not suggest that hypoxaemia had a direct effect on right ventricular myocardial function. Ten patients were also studied before and after 6 months of domiciliary oxygen (15 hours/day, 1-3 l/minute). There were no significant changes in FEV_1, FVC, systemic arterial blood pressure, PaO_2 or $PaCO_2$ after treatment. However, in spite of a fall in pulmonary arterial pressure after 6 months' domiciliary oxygen, RVEF did not change (Table IV).

Table IV. Effects of oxygen (1-3 l/min, 15 hours/day for 6 months). All values breathing room air.

	Control	6 months' oxygen	p value
FEV_1 (l)	0.60±0.04	0.50±0.04	NS
FVC (l)	1.70±0.20	1.60±0.20	NS
PaO_2 (kPa)	6.80±0.30	7.00±0.30	NS
$PaCO_2$ (kPa)	6.80±0.30	6.50±0.30	NS
Mean systemic BP (mmHg)	91.00±3.00	90.00±3.0	NS
Mean pulmonary arterial pressure (mmHg)	32.00±2.00	26.00±2.00	0.01
RVEF	0.44±0.03	0.48±0.02	NS
LVEF	0.54±0.04	0.59±0.04	NS

Right Ventricular Function in Decompensated Cor Pulmonale

Whether the clinical syndrome of oedema and raised jugular venous pressure in patients with hypoxic COPD truly represents right ventricular failure has important implications for therapy, which at present is supportive with oxygen therapy and diuretics, although ACE inhibitors and vasodilators may be contemplated in the future. It is interesting that not all patients presenting during an acute exacerbation of COPD with worsening hypoxaemia and presumably higher pulmonary arterial pressure, develop the clinical syndrome of cor pulmonale.[77]

The cause of the oedema in this syndrome remains controversial.[5,6] Although pulmonary arterial pressure is high during exacerbations of COPD and falls on recovery,[76] Khaja[25] has shown that the relationship between the right ventricular stroke work and right ventricular end-diastolic pressure is normal even in patients with right ventricular hypertrophy.

Moreover, the right ventricular maximum isovolumic development of right ventricular pressure (dp/dt) is also normal in patients with pulmonary hypertension and signs of right ventricular failure, secondary to left ventricular dysfunction.[18] We studied two groups of patients with severe hypoxic COPD, with and without oedema, but with similar levels of pulmonary arterial pressure (range 25-40 mmHg), and normal pulmonary capillary wedge pressures (mean 8±4 mmHg).[77]

Although RVEF was low (0.23±0.11) and the right ventricular end-systolic volume was higher in those with oedema suggesting decreased right ventricular contractility, this did not appear to have arisen as a result of an increase in pulmonary vascular resistance which was similar in both groups.[77]

Breathing oxygen did not change the right ventricular end-systolic pressure/ volume relationship. Cardiac output and stroke work appeared to be preserved by an adaptive mechanism resulting from a large increase in end-diastolic volume.

Right Ventricular Function and Survival

The relationship between the presence of pulmonary arterial hypertension[8] or oedema,[7] and survival in patients with COPD is well known. However, whether this represents a causal relationship is still debated. This is of more than academic interest since if cor pulmonale is a major cause of death in patients with hypoxic COPD, then treatment should be directed towards the reduction of pulmonary hypertension. In order to determine if right ventricular performance influences survival, we studied 115 patients with COPD and a wide range of disability over an average follow up period of 3 years.[78] Using a Cox's survival model we found a correlation between RVEF and survival. However RVEF was a poor predictor of survival when compared with arterial blood gas values. Indeed when the PaO_2 and $PaCO_2$ tensions were entered in the model, none of the remaining variables were significantly related to survival.

We therefore believe that RVEF, and presumably pulmonary arterial pressure are measurements of the severity of the COPD and are not causally related to survival. It appears from our data that arterial blood gas values or the degree of airflow limitation have a stronger correlation with survival than the RVEF. Indeed, in Weitzenblum's original paper[8] on the prognostic value of pulmonary arterial pressure in COPD an FEV_1 <1.2 l was as good a predictor of survival as a pulmonary arterial pressure of >20 mmHg. Our view would therefore be that patients may die with cor pulmonale, but they rarely die of it!

Right Ventricular Dimensions Measured by Magnetic Resonance Imaging (MRI)

In view of the WHO pathological definition of cor pulmonale, we studied the right ventricle by MRI using cardiac gating, in 16 patients with severe, but stable, COPD who were being assessed for domiciliary oxygen. These patients had a wide range of FEV$_1$ (0.4-1.4 l), arterial oxygen (PaO$_2$ 4.2-8.3 kPa), carbon dioxide tensions (PaCO$_2$ 4.9-8.1 kPa) and pulmonary arterial pressure (Ppa 18-46 mmHg).

We measured the right ventricular free wall volume and chamber volume and correlated these measurements with pulmonary haemodynamics measured by Swan-Ganz catheter.

There were significant correlations between the right ventricular free wall volume and the pulmonary arterial pressure (r=0.72, p<0.01) and pulmonary vascular resistance (r=0.65, p<0.01). Interestingly right ventricular free wall volume correlated with the arterial carbon dioxide tension (r=0.56, p<0.02) but not with the arterial oxygen tension. Thus this non-invasive technique can be used to measure right ventricular dimensions in life and may be used to define cor pulmonale and to study the effects on the right ventricle of therapeutic interventions, such as long-term oxygen therapy.

Oedema in Patients with Hypoxic COPD

From the data presented in this review, the increase in right ventricular end-diastolic volume which occurs in patients with COPD and oedema does not appear to be as a direct result of an increase in pulmonary arterial pressure. Thus the mechanism producing the oedema of cor pulmonale remains unclear. Several studies undertaken over 20 years ago suggest that changes in renal hormones and renal blood flow may play a central role in the development of the oedema in such patients. The most consistent observation is a reduced renal blood flow in hypoxic patients.[79-81]

Although the changes in renal blood flow are not closely related to the changes in arterial blood gas tensions which occur during recovery from an exacerbation of COPD, it seems likely that hypoxia and possibly hypercapnia may result in local renal vasoconstriction.[79] A reduction in renal blood flow might stimulate the renin/angiotensin system so retaining salt and water.

The conversion of angiotensin I to angiotensin II requires the angiotension converting enzyme, which is abundant in the pulmonary vascular endothelium. Although hypoxia has been shown to reduce the activity of this enzyme variably in peripheral blood,[82] angiotensin conversion across the pulmonary circulation in patients with COPD is not affected by oxygen therapy.[83]

Atrial natriuretic peptide, which is stored in the granules of both atria appears to be an important hormone in salt and water balance.

Recently Burghuber[84] found higher levels on ANP in the central as opposed to the peripheral circulation in patients with COPD. The level of plasma ANP correlated with the right atrial pressure, suggesting atrial distension caused the release of ANP. However, surprisingly, this relationship was present within a group of patients with normal right atrial pressures. We have also recently measured ANP across the pulmonary circulation in 11 patients with COPD, studied when clinically stable, and in addition have made measurements serially in peripheral blood in twelve patients during exacerbations of COPD. We were unable to confirm Burghuber's observation that ANP was higher in central, rather than peripheral blood. However, we also found a correlation between plasma ANP and the right atrial pressure ($r = 0.7$ $p<0.05$). However, an even better correlation was present between the right ventricular end-diastolic volume, measured by magnetic resonance imaging ($r = 0.8$, $p<0.01$) and plasma ANP, which we believe relates to right ventricular and hence right atrial distension. Breathing oxygen 2 l/minute by nasal prongs, did not change pulmonary haemodynamics nor the level of atrial natriuretic peptide. Patients with acute exacerbations of COPD, particularly those with oedema had higher values of ANP than those without oedema, and again breathing oxygen for 1 hour did not change plasma ANP. However, the mean change in body weight during the first 3 days of the admission correlated with the change in plasma ANP over the same period ($r = 0.8$, $p<0.05$). The fact that high levels of a natriuretic peptide are found in the presence of peripheral oedema in patients with COPD requires further study. Moreover, the role of ANP as a therapy for such patients is as yet unclear.

References

1. Registrar General of Scotland. *Annual Report*, Edinburgh, HM Stationery Office, Edinburgh, 1982
2. World Health Organization. Chronic cor pulmonale. A report of the expert committee. Circulation 1963; 27:594-598
3. Fishman A.P.: State of the art: chronic cor pulmonale. Am. Rev. Respir. Dis. 1976; 114:775-794
4. Magee F., Wright J.L., Wiggs B.R., Pare P.D., Hogg J.C.: Pulmonary vascular structure and function in chronic obstructive pulmonary disease. Thorax 1988; 43:183-189
5. Richens J.M., Howard P.: Oedema in cor pulmonale. Clin. Sci. 1982; 62:255-259
6. Morrison D.A.: Pulmonary hypertension in chronic obstructive pulmonary disease. The right ventricular hypothesis. Chest 1987; 92:387-388
7. Renzetti A.D., McClement J.H., Litt B.D.: The veterans administration co-operative study of pulmonary function III. Mortality in relation to respiratory function in chronic obstructive pulmonary disease. Am. J. Med. 1966; 41:115-119
8. Weitaenblum E., Hirth C., Ducolone A., Mirholm R., Rasahalinjonahary J., Ehrhart M.: Prognostic value of pulmonary artery pressure in chronic obstructive pulmonary disease. Thorax 1981; 36:752-758
9. Arcilla R.A., Tsai P., Thilenus O., Ranninger K.: Angiographic method for volume estimation of the right and left ventricles. Chest 1971; 60:446-454
10. Gentzler R., Briselli M., Gault J.: Angiographic estimation of the right ventricular volume in man. Circulation 1974; 4:1-55
11. Fishman A.P.: Cor pulmonale: General aspects. In: Fishman A.P. (Ed.) *Pulmonary diseases and disorders*. New York: McGraw-Hill 1980; 853-882
12. Laks M.M., Garner D., Swan H.J.C.: Volumes and compliances measured simultaneously in the

right and left ventricles of the dog. Circ. Res. 1967; 20:565-569

13. Abel F.L.: Effects of alterations in peripheral resistance on left ventricular function. Proc. Soc. Exp. Biol. Med. 1965; 120:52-56

14. McFadden E.R., Braunwald E.: Cor pulmonale and pulmonary thromboembolism. In: Braunwald E. (Ed.) *Heart disease a textbook of cardiovascular medicine*. Philadelphia, WB Saunders 1980; 1643-1680

15. Bishop J.M., Cross K.W.: Use of other physiological variables to predict pulmonary arterial pressure in patients with chronic respiratory disease: a multicentre study. Eur. Heart J. 1981; 2:509-517

16. Weitzenblum E., Loiseau A., Hirth C., et al.: Course of pulmonary haemodynamics in patients with chronic obstructive pulmonary disease. Chest 1979; 75:656-662

17. Schrijen F., Uffholtz H., Polu J.M., et al.: Pulmonary and systemic haemodynamic evaluation of chronic bronchitis. Am. Rev. Respir. Dis. 1978; 117:25-31

18. Stein P.D., Saggah N.H., Ande D.T., Marzilli M.: Performance of the failing and non-failing right ventricle of patients with pulmonary hypertension. Am. J. Cardiol. 1979; 44:1050-1055

19. Wagenvoort C.A., Wagenvoort N.: Primary pulmonary hypertension: a pathological study of the lung vessels in 156 clinically diagnosed cases. Circulation 1970; 42:1163-1184

20. Berglund E.: Haemodynamics of the right ventricle in chronic lung disease. Bull. Physiol.-pathol., Resp. 1972; 8:1417-1422

21. Boushy J.F., North L.B.: Haemodynamic changes in chronic obstructive pulmonary disease. Chest 1977; 72:565-570

22. Burrows B., Kettel L.J., Niden A.H., Rabinowitz M., Diere C.F.: Patterns of cardiovascular dysfunction in chronic obstructive lung disease. New Engl. J. Med. 1972; 286:912-918

23. Fishman A.P.: Hypoxia and its effects on the pulmonary circulation. How and where it acts. Circ. Res. 1976; 38:221-231

24. Jezek V., Schrigen F., Sadoul P.: Right ventricular function and pulmonary haemodynamics during exercise in patients with chronic obstructive broncho-pulmonary disease. Cardiology 1973; 58:20-31

25. Khaja F., Parker J.O.: Right and left ventricular performance in chronic obstructive lung disease. Am. Heart J. 1971; 82:319-327

26. Harris P., Heath D.: The human pulmonary circulation: its form and function in health and disease. Edinburgh, Churchill Livingstone, 1986

27. Bistow J.D., Morris J.F., Kloster F.E.: Haemodynamics of cor pulmonale. Proc. Cardiovasc. Dis. 1966; 9:239-258

28. Borden C.W., Wilson R.H., Ebert R.V., et al.: Pulmonary hypertension in chronic pulmonary emphysema. Am. J. med. 1950; 8.701-709

29. Kline L.E., Crawford M.T., MacDonald W.J., Schelbert H., O'Rourke R.A., Moser K.M.: Non-invasive assessment of left ventricular performance in patients with chronic obstructive pulmonary disease. Chest 1977; 72:558-564

30. Mounsey J.P.D., Titzman L.W., Selverstone N.J., et al.: Circulatory changes in severe pulmonary emphysema. Br. Heart J. 1952; 14:153-172

31. Williams J.F., Behuke R.H.: The effect of pulmonary emphysema upon cardiopulmonary haemodynamics at rest and during exercise. Ann. Int. Med. 1964; 60:824-842

32. Reedy T., Chapman C.B.: Measurement of right ventricular volume by cineangiofluorography. Am. Heart J. 1963; 66:221-225

33. Xue Q.F., MacNee W., Flenley D.C., Hannan W.J., Muir A.L.: Can right ventricular performance be assessed by gated equilibrium ventriculography? Thorax 1983; 38:486-493

34. Maddahi J., Bermon D.S., Matsuoka D.T., Waxman A.D., Stankus K.E., Foorester J.S., Swan

H.J.C.: A new technique for assessing right ventricular ejection fraction using rapid multiple gated equilibrium cardiac blood pool scintigraphy. Circulation 1979; 60:581-589

35. Wathen C.G., Hannan W.J., Flenley D.C., Muir A.L.: Reproducibility of radionuclide right ventricular ejection fraction (RVEF) in chronic bronchitis and emphysema (COLD). Clin. Sci. 1988; 74 (Suppl 18): 60P.

36. Ellis J.H., Kirch D., Steele P.P.: Right ventricular ejection fraction in severe chronic airway obstruction (Abstr.). Chest 1977; 71:(Suppl) 281-282

37. Olvey S.K., Reduto L.A., Stevens P.M., et al.: First pass radionuclide asessment of right and left ventricular ejection fraction in COPD. Chest 1980; 78:4-9

38. Berger H.J., Matthay R.A., Loke J., Marshall R.C., Gottschalk A., Zaret B.L.: Assessment of cardiac performance with quantitative radionuclide angiography: right ventricular ejection fraction with reference to findings in chronic obstructive pulmonary disease. Am. J. Cardiol. 1978; 41:897-905

39. Matthay R.A., Berger H.J.: Cardiovascular performance in chronic obstructive pulmonary diseases. Med. Clin. N. Am. 1981; 65:489-520

40. Slutsky R., Hooper W., Gerber K., et al.: Assessment of right ventricular function at rest and during exercise in patients with coronary artery disease. Am. J. Cardiol. 1980; 45:63-71

41. Mathur P., Bowles P., Pugsley S., et al.: Effect of digoxin on right ventricular function in severe chronic airflow obstruction. Ann. Intern. Med. 1981; 95:283-288

42. Hooper W.W., Slutsky R.A., Kocienski D.E.: Right and left ventricular response to subcutaneous terbutaline in patients with chronic obstructive pulmonary disease: radionuclide angiography, assessment of cardiac size and function. Am. Heart J. 1982; 104:1027-1032

43. Dahlstrom J.A.: Simultaneous assessment of right ventricular ejection fraction and central haemodynamics at rest and during exercise in patients with pulmonary hypertension. Clinical Physiology 1983; 3:267-279

44. Erickson A.D., Golden W.A., Calunch B.S., Donat W.E., Kalmmerlen J.T.: Acute effects of phlebotomy on right ventricular size and performance in polycythemic patients with chronic obstructive pulmonary disease. Am. J. Cardiol. 1983; 163-166

45. Brown S.E., Pakron F.J., Milne N., et al.: Effects of digoxin on exercise capacity and right ventricular function during exercise in chronic airflow obstruction. Chest 1984; 85:187-191

46. Tuxien D.V., Powles A.C.P., Mathur P.N., Pugsley S.O., Campbell E.J.M.: Detrimental effects of hydralazine in patients with chronic airflow obstruction and pulmonary hypertension. A controlled haemodynamic and radionuclide study. Am. Rev. Respir. Dis. 1984; 129:388-395

47. Brent B.N., Mahler D., Matthay R.A., Berger H.J., Zaret B.L.: Non-invasive diagnosis of pulmonary arterial hypertension in chronic obstructive pulmonary disease: right ventricular ejection fraction at rest. Am. J. Cardiol. 1984; 53:1349-1353

48. Burghuber O.C., Bergmann H.: Right ventricular contractility in chronic obstructive pulmonary disease. Respiration 1988; 53:1-12 .

49. Morrison D., Goloman S., Wright A.L., et al.: The effect of pulmonary hypertension on systolic function of the right ventricle. Chest 1983; 84:250-257

50. Reduto L.A., Berger H.J., Cohen L.S., Gottschalk A., Zaret B.L.: Sequential radionuclide assessment of left and right ventricular performance after acute myocardial infarction. Ann. Int. Med. 1978; 89.441-447

51. Tobinick E., Schelelbert H.R., Henning et al.: Right ventricular ejection fraction in patients with acute anterior and inferior myocardial infarction assessed by radionuclide angiography. Circulation 1978; 1078-1084

52. MacNee W., Xue Q.F., Hannan W.J., Flenley D.C., Adie C.J., Muir A.L.: Assessment by radionuclide angiography of right and left ventricular function in chronic bronchitis and

emphysema. Thorax 1983; 38:494-500

53. Berger H.J., Matthay R.A., Davies R.A., Zaret B.L., Gottschalk A.: Comparison of exercise right ventricular performance in chronic obstructive pulmonary disease and coronary artery disease: non-invasive assessment by quantitative radionuclide angiocardiography. Invest. Radiol. 1979; 14:342-353

54. MacNee W., Morgan A.D., Wathen C.G., Muir A.L., Flenley D.C.: Right ventricular performance during exercise in chronic obstructive pulmonary disease: the effect of oxygen. Respiration 1985; 48:206-211

55. Gould G., MacNee W., McLean A., Warren P.M., Redpath A., Best J.J.K., Lamb D., Flenley D.C.: CT measurement of lung density in life can quantitate distal airspace enlargment - an essential defining feature of human emphysema. Am. Rev. Respir. Dis. 1988; 137:380-392

56. Biernacki W., Gould G.A., Whyte K.F., Flenley D.C.: Pulmonary haemodynamics, gas exchange, and the severity of emphysema as assessed by quantitative CT scan in chronic bronchitis and emphysema. Am. Rev. Respir. Dis. 1989; 139:1509-1515

57. Winzelberg G.G., Boucher C.A., Pohost G.M., et al.: Right ventricular function in aortic and mitral valve disease. Relation of gated first pass radionuclide angiography to clinic and haemodynamic findings. Chest 1981; 79:520-528

58. Korr K.S., Grandsman E.J., Winkler M.L., Schulman R.S., Bough E.W.: Haemodynamic correlates of right ventricular ejection fraction measured with gated radionuclide angiography. Am. J. Cardiol. 1982; 49:71-77

59. Friedman B.J., Holman B.L.: Scintigraphic prediction of pulmonary arterial systolic pressure by regional right ventricular ejection fraction during the second half of systole. Am. J. Cardiol. 1978; 50: 1114-1119

60. Morrison D.A., Sorenson S., Caldwell J., Wright A.L., Ritchie J., Kennedy J.W., et al.: The normal right ventricular response to supine exercise. Chest 1982; 82:686:691

61. Brent B.N., Berger H.J., Matthay R.A., Mahler R., Pytlik M., Zaret B.L.: Physiologic correlates of right ventricular ejection fraction in chronic obstructive pulmonary disease. A combined radionuclide haemodynamic study. Am. J. Cardiol. 1982; 50:255-262

62. Mahler D.A., Brent B.N., Loke J., Zaret B.L., Matthay R.A.: Right ventricular performance and central circulatory haemodynamics during upright exercise in patients with chronic obstructive pulmonary disease. Am. Rev. Respir. Dis. 1984; 130:722-729

63. Burghuber O., Bergman H., Silberbauer K., Hofer R.: Right ventricular performance in chronic airflow obstruction. Respiration 1984; 45:124-130

64. Biernacki W., MacNee W., Flenley D.C., Muir A.L.: The effect of pulmonary hypertension on right ventricular function in patients with chronic obstructive pulmonary disease. Chest 1988; 94:1149-1175

65. Caro C.G., Pedley T.J., Schroter R.C., Seed W.A.: *The mechanics of the circulation.* Oxford: Oxford University Press, 1981; 213-214

66. Braunwald E., Sonnenblick E.K., Ross J.Jr.: Contraction of the normal heart. In: Braunwald E. (Ed.) *Heart disease.* Philadelphia, WB Saunders 1984; 409-447

67. Permutt S.: Relation between pulmonary arterial pressure and pleural pressure during the acute asthmatic attack. Chest 1973; (Suppl) 63:25-28

68. Gunther S., Grossman W.: Determinants of ventricular function in pressure and pleural pressure during the acute asthmatic attack. Chest 1973; (Suppl) 63:25-28

68. Gunther S., Grossman W.: Determinants of ventricular function in pressure overload hypertrophy in man. Circulation 1979; 679-688

69. Sagawa K.: The end-systolic pressure volume relation of the ventricle; definition, modifications and clinical use. Circulation 1981; 63:1223-1227

134

70. Sagawa K.: The ventricular pressure volume diagram revisited. Circulation Res. 1978; 677-686
71. Grossman W., Braunwald E., Man T., McLaurin L.P., Green L.H.: Contractile state of the left ventricle in man as evaluated from end-systolic pressure volume relations. Circulation 1977; 56:845-852
72. Suga H., Sagawa K., Shoukas A.A.: Load independence of the instantaneous pressure volume ratio of the canine left ventricle and effects of epinephrine and heart rate on the ratio. Circ. Res. 1973; 32:314-321
73. Braunwald E., Sonnenblick E.H., Ross J.Jr.: Contraction of the normal heart. In: Braunwald E. (Ed.) *Heart Disease*. Philadelphia, WB Saunders 1984; 409-447
74. Marsh J.D., Green L.H., Wynne J., Cohn P.F., Grossman W.: Left ventricular end-systolic pressure-dimension and stress-length relations in normal human subjects. Am. J. Cardiol. 1979; 44:1311-1317
75. MacNee W., Wathen C.G., Hannan W.J., Flenley D.C., Muir A.L.: The effects of pirbuterol and sodium nitroprusside on pulmonary haemodynamics in hypoxic cor pulmonale. Br. Med. J. 1983; 287:1169-1172
76. Abraham A.S., Cole R.B., Green I.D., Hedworth-Whitty R.B., Clarke S.W., Bishop J.M.: Factors contributing to the reversible pulmonary hypertension in patients with acute respiratory failure studied by serial observations during recovery. Circ. Res. 1969; 26:51-60
77. MacNee W., Wathen C.G., Flenley D.C., Muir A.L.: The effects of controlled oxygen therapy on ventricular function in patients with stable and decompensated cor pulmonale. Am. Rev. Respir. Dis. 1988; 137:1289-1295
78. France A.J., Prescott R.J., Biernacki W., Muir A.L., MacNee W.: Does right ventricular function predict survival in patients with chronic obstructive lung disease? Thorax 1988; 43:621-626
79. Aber G.M., Bayley J.J., Bishop J.M.: Inter-relationships between renal and cardiac function and respiratory gas exchange in obstructive airways disease. Clin. Sci. 1963; 25:159-170
80. Platts M.M., Hammond J.D.S., Stuart-Harris C.H.: A study of cor pulmonale in patients with chronic bronchtitis. Quart. J. Med. 1960; 29:559-574
81. Stuart-Harris C.H., MacKinnon J., Hammond J.D.S., Smith W.D.: The renal circulation in chronic pulmonary disease and pulmonary heart failure. Quart. J. Med. 1956; 25:389-405
82. Milledge J.S., Catley D.M.: Renin, aldosterone and converting enzyme: exercise and acute hypoxia in humans. J. Appl. Physiol. 1982; 52:320-323
83. Neilly J.B., Clark C.J., Tweddel A., et al.: Transpulmonary angiotension II formation in patients with chronic stable cor pulmonale. Am. Rev. Respir. Dis. 1987; 135:891-895
84. Burghuber O.C., Hartter E., Punzengruber C., Weissel M., Woloszczk W.: Human atrial natriuretic peptide secretion in pre-capillary pulmonary hypertension: clinical study in patients with COPD and interstitial fibrosis. Chest 1988; 93:31-37

11. Right Ventricular Contractility is Preserved and Preload Increased in Patients with Chronic Obstructive Pulmonary Disease and Pulmonary Artery Hypertension

O.C. BURGHUBER

Second Medical Department, University of Vienna, Austria

Introduction

Pulmonary hypertension and right heart failure are major causes of death in patients with COPD.[1-3] The effect of pulmonary artery hypertension on right ventricular function is by no means clear. In the past, quantification of right ventricular function has been difficult because of the complex geometry of the right ventricle. Non-invasive radionuclide studies by measuring RVEF have recently indicated preclinical right ventricular dysfunction in patients with COPD. We[4] and others[5,6], however, convincingly have shown that RVEF appears to be highly dependent on afterload, thus raising the question concerning its use as a parameter of overall right ventricular function.

We therefore addressed the issue of right ventricular function in a group of 24 patients with COPD with and without pulmonary hypertension using a combined radionuclide-haemodynamic approach. Estimations of RVEF by radionuclide method and stroke volume index (SVI) by thermodilution were obtained simultaneously and right ventricular volumes were derived. From these and the measured pressures in the right heart, right ventricular end-systolic pressure-volume relations were calculated as a means of defining right ventricular intrinsic contractility independent of loading conditions.

Materials and Methods

Population and lung function: 24 white males with COPD, selected from our outpatient clinic, were included in this study after obtaining informed consent. Criteria of selection of patients for the study were as follows: presence of acutely non-reversible airflow limitation as determined by a FEV_1/VC ratio of less than 65% and IGV/TLC ratio of more than 50%, absence of right sided heart failure and absence of left ventricular disease, assessed by history, physical examination, ECG and two dimensional echocardiography (Sonolayer, SSH-60 a, Toshiba).

Pulmonary function tests were performed using standard spirometric and body plethysmographic techniques.[7]

Right heart catheterization

Patients were examined at noon time, supine and fasting. Swan Ganz balloon directed catheters (American Edwards Laboratories, model 93A/100/5F) were inserted percutaneously into an antecubital vein.

Pressures were recorded continuously using transducers (Hewlett-Packard HP 1290) coupled to a pressure monitor (Hewlett-Packard HP 7834 2A) using a channel recorder (Hellige Multiscriptor EK 36).

The following pressures (in mmHg), were recorded: mean right atrial pressure (pra), right ventricular end-diastolic pressure (RVEDP), systolic (Pap_s), diastolic (Pap_d), mean (Pap_m) pulmonary artery pressure, and pulmonary capillary wedge pressure (PCWP).

Cardiac output was determined in triplicate by the thermodilution technique (Computer Model 9528, Edwards Laboratory). Blood gases were measured on a radiometer ABL blood gas analyser (ABL Acid Base Laboratory; Radiometer, Copenhagen).

Radionuclide technique

Equilibrium radionuclide angiograms were obtained in the anterior position according to standard techniques using [81m]krypton as a tracer. The procedure has been described in detail previously.[8]

The right ventricular ejection fraction (RVEF) was calculated from the background corrected time activity curve of the right ventricle, using the formula RVEF (%) = ED-ES/ED x 100, where ED and ES represents background corrected counts in end-diastole and end-systole, respectively. Normal value for RVEF in our laboratory was 58% (range 45%-67%). From the haemodynamic data alone and in conjunction with RVEF the following variables were derived:

- Cardiac Index (CI l/min/m^2) = CO/body surface area
- Pulmonary Vascular Resistance (PVR; dyn. sec. cm^{-5}) = PAP$_m$ - PCWP/CO
- Stroke Volume Index (SVI; ml/beat/min) = CI/heart rate
- Right ventricular end-diastolic volume index (RVEDVI; ml/m^2) = SVI/RVEF
- Right ventricular end-systolic volume index (RVESVI; ml/m^2) = RVEDVI - SVI

The ratio of right ventricular end-systolic pressure to right ventricular end-systolic volume index (RVESP/RVESVI; mmHg/mml/m²) has been shown to be a sensitive parameter in assessing contractility independent of systolic loading conditions.[9,10]

Statistics

Data are expressed as mean ± SEM unless stated differently. Paired and unpaired Student t tests were used to compare results within and between groups respectively. Regression and correlation methods were used when looking for the relationship among selected variables. $p<0.05$ was considered significant.

Results

COPD patients were divided into two groups, according whether or not resting pulmonary artery hypertension ($Pap_m > 20$ mmHg) was present. Based on this parameter 13 patients had pulmonary artery hypertension (Group 1) and 11 patients (Group 2) had normal resting pulmonary artery pressures ($Pap_m < 20$ mmHg). By definition, Pap_m was higher in group 1 (30.5±2.6 mmHg) than in group 2 (15.3±1.0 mmHg; $p<0.001$) as was mean pulmonary vascular resistance (290±25 dyn.sec.cm⁻⁵ vs. 156±33 dyn.sec.cm⁻⁵, $p<0.001$).

The average age (63.1 ± 11.8 years vs. 61.6 ± 6.1 years), height (171.1 ± 6.8 cm vs. 170 ± 5.6 cm) and weight (75.1 ± 16.1 kg vs. 74.9 ± 9.3 kg) were almost identical in the COPD patients with or without pulmonary artery hypertension.

The most striking difference in pulmonary function and blood gas analysis between the two groups was a much lower arterial oxygen tension (PaO_2) in patients with pulmonary artery hypertension (60.1±2.3 mmHg), compared with the PaO_2 of patients without pulmonary artery hypertension (69.6±2.2 mmHg, $p<0.001$). In addition the group of patients with pulmonary artery hypertension exhibited a lower vital capacity (2.8±0.9 l vs. 3.5±0.8 l $p<0.05$), whereas the other lung function parameters did not differ between the two groups.

All patients studied had normal left ventricular function (PCWP: 7.2±1.1 mmHg; CI: 3.5±0.1 l/min/m²) and normal mean right atrial pressures (pra: 4.5 ± 1.3 mmHg).

Figure 1 shows mean values of RVEF and Table I mean RVEF, right ventricular volume indices and pressure-volume relations derived from haemodynamic data in conjunction with RVEF. Mean RVEF was normal in group 2 and significantly higher than in group 1($p<0.001$).

Mean SVI was normal in all COPD patients and did not differ between the groups. Mean RVEDVI was normal in group 2 (normal range: 80-100 ml/m²) but increased in group 1 patients, the difference being statistically significant ($p<0.05$). RVESVI was also significantly higher in patients with pulmonary artery hypertension ($p<0.05$).

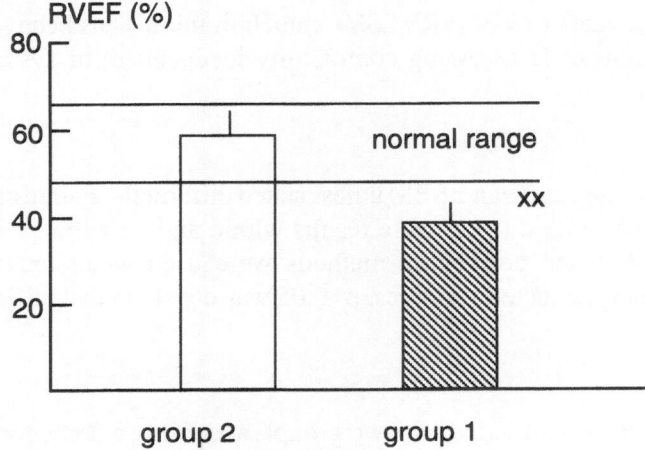

Fig. 1. Mean ± SEM of right ventricular ejection fraction (RVEF) in COPD patients with (Group 1) and without (Group 2) pulmonary artery hypertension; ** p < 0.001; group 1 *vs.* group 2.

Table I. Right ventricular ejection fraction, right ventricular volume indices and pressure-volume relation in COPD patients with or without pulmonary artery hypertension (mean ±SEM); for abbreviations see text

	COPD patients without PH (n = 11)	COPD patients with PH (n = 13)
RVEF (%)	55.10 ± 4.10	44.40 ± 3.00**
SVI (ml/m²)	47.00 ± 4.50	38.00 ± 2.80
RVEDVI (ml/m²)	85.30 ± 9.40	115.00 ± 7.30*
RVESVI (ml/m²)	38.30 ± 7.40	77.00 ± 11.60*
RVESP/RVESVI (mmHg/ml/m²)	0.83 ± 0.13	0.67 ± 0.08

** p < 0.001, * p < 0.05; with *vs.* without pulmonary artery hypertension

Finally, pressure-volume relation (RVESP/RVESVI), the parameter of right ventricular intrinsic contractility averaged 0.73 ± 0.07 mmHg/ml/m² and was not different in the two groups studied. RVEF strongly correlated with parameters of afterload (Pap_m: r=0.73; p<0.001; PVR: r=0.69; p<0.001) and weakly with the parameter of preload (RVEDVI: r=0.49; p<0.05) but did not correlate with the parameter of intrinsic right ventricular contractility (RVESP/RVESVI: r=0.39; n.s.).

Discussion

The main finding of this study is that despite a decreased right ventricular ejection fraction, overall right ventricular function and in particular right ventricular contractility, is well preserved even in COPD patients with pulmonary artery hypertension. Therefore, the right ventricular ejection fraction seems to be not a good parameter of overall right ventricular function and/or contractility in these patients. The increased right ventricular end-diastolic volume index indicates that the major mechanism of maintaining stroke volume upon increased afterload conditions appears to be the Frank-Starling mechanism.

The infusion of the inert gas [81m]krypton into the right heart seems to be an ideal method of determining RVEF, combining the advantages of the methods using ^{99m}Tc without their shortcomings. The main advantage is that the tracer does not reach the left heart, since it is completely exhaled on its passage through the lung.

The right ventricle is thus imaged without superimposition of the left heart. In addition, this method has been shown to be valid and highly reproducible for this purpose,[11,12] and the values obtained are similar to those reported by others using [99m]Tc.[13,14] By combining this method with an independent measurement of right ventricular stroke volume by thermodilution techniques, we were able to calculate right ventricular end-diastolic and end-systolic volumes, which further allowed us to calculate right ventricular pressure-volume relations in order to examine right ventricular contractility independent of loading conditions.

Using these techniques, the present study confirms our previous observation,[4] that RVEF is diminished in COPD patients with pulmonary artery hypertension and that this parameter is highly dependent on afterload conditions, in that inverse correlations between RVEF and either Pap_m or PVR were noted. In contrast, no correlation between RVEF and overall right ventricular function as assessed by SVI and CI, or right ventricular contractility as assessed by pressure-volume relations, could be demonstrated. Thus it appears that altered right ventricular afterload was a major factor modulating RVEF in our COPD patients.

Therefore, the reduction in RVEF in our COPD patients did not necessarily imply altered intrinsic myocardial contractility. In order to better evaluate the response of the right ventricle to increased afterload stress, we compared various parameters of right ventricular function in a homogeneous group of COPD patients with and without pulmonary artery hypertension.

The degree of obstructive lung disease was almost identical in the two groups, whereas PaO_2 was significantly higher in COPD patients without pulmonary artery hypertension, suggesting hypoxic pulmonary vasoconstriction being a major cause of pulmonary artery hypertension in our COPD patients.

Increase in preload and/or increase in intrinsic myocardial contractility are the two compensatory mechanisms known to be available for the right ventricle to keep a normal stroke volume in face of an increased afterload stress. In our COPD patients with pulmonary artery hypertension in whom stroke volume was normal, RVEDVI, the best parameter of right ventricular preload[15] was higher than normal and higher than in patients without pulmonary artery hypertension. Thus, it seems that in our patients, one mechanism by which the right ventricle - facing increased afterload - maintained stroke volume was an increase in preload reflecting the Frank-Starling mechanism.

The ability of the right ventricle to respond to an increase in afterload by increasing its contractility, as it is known from the left ventricle, is probably limited by the thinness of the right ventricular free wall. This idea is in agreement with our finding that the right ventricular pressure-volume relation, a sensitive parameter in assessing contractility independent of loading conditions,[9,16] was not higher in patients with pulmonary artery hypertension. Thus, preload augmentation seem to be the main mechanism in maintaining stroke volume when afterload is increased, whereas increase in contractility does not play a major role.

In summary, pulmonary artery hypertension complicating COPD is characterized by an increase in right ventricular preload which may be the major mechanism to maintain adequate flow from the right to the left ventricle. The decreased RVEF observed in these patients is primarily due to increased afterload conditions rather than an indication of right ventricular myocardial dysfunction. In a stable condition, right ventricular contractility seems to be well maintained in COPD patients even with pulmonary artery hypertension.

References

1. Mitchel R.S., Webb N.C., Filey G.F.: Chronic obstructive broncho-pulmonary disease III. Factors influencing prognosis. Am. Rev. Resp. Dis. 1964; 89:878-896
2. Traver G.A., Cline M.G., Burrow: Predictors of mortality in chronic obstructive pulmonary disease. Am. Rev. Resp. Dis. 1979; 119:895-902
3. Higgin M.W., Keller J.W., Becker M: An index of risk for obstructive airway disease. Am. Rev. Resp. Dis. 1982; 125:144-152
4. Burghuber O.C., Bergman H., Silberbauer K., Höfer R.: Right ventricular performance in chronic airflow obstruction. Respiration 1984; 45:124-130
5. Brent B.N., Berger H.J., Matthay R.A., Mahler D., Rytlik L., Zaret B.L.: Physiologic correlate of right ventricular ejection fraction in chronic obstructive pulmonary disease: a combined radionuclide-hemodynamic study. Am. J. Cardiol. 1982; 50:255-262
6. Korr K.S., Gandsman E.J., Winkler M.L., Shulman R.S., Bough E.W.: Hemodynamic correlates of right ventricular ejection fraction measured with gated radionuclide angiography. Am. J. Cardiol. 1982; 49:71-77
7. Burghuber O.C., Hartter E., Punzengruber C.H., Weissel M., Woloszczuk: Human atrial natriuretic peptide secretion in precapillary pulmonary hypertension. Chest 1988; 93:31-37
8. Burghuber O.C., Salzer Muhar U., Bergman H., Götz M.: Right ventricular performance and hemodynamics in adolescent and adult patients with cystic fibrosis. Eur. J. Pediatr. 1988; 148:187-192

9. Dehmer G.L., Corbett J., Hillis L.D., Lewis S.E., Parkey R.W., Willerson J.T.: The end syst. P/V index: a sensitive parameter for the scintigraphic detection of left ventricular in patients with coronary artery disease. Circulation 1980; 62:4-12

10. Suga H.:, Sagawa K.: Instantaneous pressure-volume relationship and their ratio in the excised, supported canine left ventricle. Circ. Res. 1974; 35:117-124

11. Nestaval A., Kidery J., Fridl P., Oppelt A., Jandova R., Widimsky J.: Radionuclide ventriculography of the right ventricle in diseases involving the heart. Prog. Resp. Res. 1985; 20:117-125

12. Wong D.F., Natarajan T.K., Summer W., Tibits P.A., Beck T., Koller D.: Right ventricular ejection fraction measured by first pass intravenous krypton 81m: reprodicibility and comparison with Tc 99m. Am. J. Cardiol. 1985; 56:776-780

13. Brent B.N., Berger H.J., Matthay R.A., Mahler D., Rytlik L., Zaret B.L.: Physiologic correlates of right ventricular ejection fraction in chronic obstructive pulmonary disease: A combined radionuclide-hemodynamic study. Am. J. Cardiol. 1982; 50:255-262

14. Korr K.S., Gandsman E.J., Winkler M.L., Shulman R.S., Bough E.W.: Hemodynamic correlates of right ventricular ejection fraction measured by gated radionuclide angiography. Am. J. Cardiol. 1982; 49:71-77

15. Mahler D.A., Brent B.N., Loke J., Zaret B.L., Matthay R.A.: Right ventricular performance and central hemodynamics during upright exercise in patients with chronic obstructive pulmonary disease. Am. Rev. Resp. Dis. 1984; 130:722-729

16. Sibbald W.J., Driedger A.A.: Right ventricular function in acute disease state: pathophysiologic considerations. Crit. Care Med. 1983; 11:339-346

12. The Right Ventricular Volumes and Function by Two-dimensional Echocardiography and Right Ventricular Angiography

P. Niederle, V. Ježek, J. Ježkova, A. Michaljanic

Institute of Physiological Regulations, Czechoslovak Academy of Sciences, Prague, Czechoslovakia

Information concerning right ventricular (RV) function is worthwhile in practice not only in cases with isolated right heart involvement, but also in the advanced stages of left ventricular failure.

The principal problem limiting the use of any method of investigation is the RV anatomy. Even the normal right ventricle has a complex and irregular shape due to non-uniform trabeculations, a separate infundibulum and variations in shape with altered loading conditions.[7]

Despite these difficulties, some angiographic studies have shown that RV volume can be accurately assessed from the projections of that ventricle in two perpendicular planes[2] and even from a single plane RV cine-angiographic image.[3] Echocardiographic attempts to determine RV volumes have appeared more recently and to date, there have been a small number of studies dealing with this topic.[1,4,5,8,12,15,16]

We were attracted to this field because of two major reasons:

1. the clinical need to evaluate the changes in RV function non-invasively;
2. the extremely favourable results of two model studies published by Weyman's group in 1984 and 1985[8,7] and the very simple approach to RV function assessment described by Kaul in 1984.[6]

The object of the present study was to test the reliability of several approaches to RV volume and/or function estimation employing two-dimensional echocardiography and to recommend the most promising method for further clinical testing.

In addition we wanted to study the influence of tricuspid regurgitation on RV function.

Patients and Methods

The investigated group consisted of 44 consecutive patients (23 male, 21 female; mean age 52.1±9.1; range 31-75 years) undergoing right heart catheterization including RV angiography. Due to the poor two-dimensional echocardiographic visualization, studies of a further 10 were considered unsatisfactory and therefore rejected. The details are listed in methodology. The review of proved clinical diagnosis in our patients was as follows:

A. *primary left heart involvement:*
- rheumatic valvular lesion   24
- coronary artery disease   4
- dilated cardiomyopathy   2
- constrictive pericarditis   1
  (initial stage)

B. *primary right heart involvement:*
- congenital atrial septal defect   5
- chronic lung disease   7
- primary pulmonary hypertension   1

In every patient a single plane RV cine-angiography in right anterior oblique projection was performed, mostly following echocardiography after a one week interval. The single-plane Ferlinz formula was applied in RV volume calculation.[3]

$$V = \frac{0.4\ A^2}{L} + 3.9 \quad (V = \text{volume}, A = \text{area}, L = \text{long axis}).$$

In 18 out of 44 patients tricuspid insufficiency was detected by RV angiography and echocardiography as well. Using an angiographic classification with four grades, regurgitation of grade I was present in 7 cases and grades II and III degree in 6 and 5 cases, respectively.[11]

Echocardiography

Echocardiographic examination was performed using an A.T.L. MK 600 mechanical sector scanner (U.S.A.) with 3 MHz transducer. The images were retained on standard video-tape recorder (Panasonic) at 60 frames for later playback analysis. A calibration grid was recorded simultaneously.

For RV evaluation we have chosen orthogonal planes corresponding to the apical

4-chamber and the subcostal RV outflow tract projections. Both planes can be easily obtained using internal echocardiographic references. From the practical point of view we have divided the quality of echocardiographic images into four categories: excellent, good, fair, and unsatisfactory.

Out of the initial 54 studies, 6 were considered excellent, 26 good, 12 fair and 10 unsatisfactory. Thus the overall success rate was 82%. The 10 excluded echocardiographic studies exhibited no specific predisposition to any disease. For RV volumes and/or function assessment, three separate methods were selected:

1. An area-length method

The RV cavity area was evaluated from the apical 4-chamber view A_{4ch} and the measurement of the long RV axis was performed in the subcostal short-axis cross-section L_{sc} (Fig. 1).

The recorded video tracings were digitized using a Cardio 200 computer (Kontron, F.R.G.). The RV cavity contours were traced by light-pen and an appropriate computer program applied for area and long axis calculation. The mean of at least three separate area and length measurements was considered as representative. The end-diastolic RV images were identified from the R peak of simultaneously recorded ECGs and end-systolic images were represented by the smallest RV cavity contours during the T wave descent.

The following formula for volume calculation was employed: $V = 2 (A_{4ch} \times L_{sc})$[3,4,8]

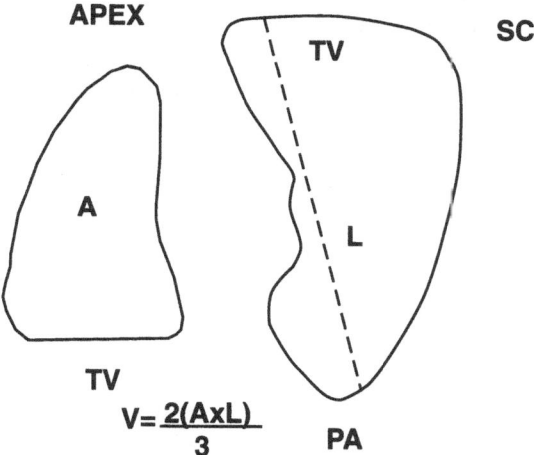

Fig. 1. The contours of RV area as obtained from apical 4-chamber v ew and subcostal RV outflow tract projection (dotted line represents the RV long axis). The original formula by Levine et al.[8] is given at the bottom. (V = volume, A = area of the 4-chamber RV image, L = RV long axis)

The ejection fraction (EF) was calculated as: $EF = \dfrac{EDV - ESV}{EDV}$

(EDV = end-diastolic volume, ESV = end-systolic volume). The described procedure was performed in all 44 patient studies.

2. Method applying Simpson's rule

The areas of both aforementioned RV images (apical and subcostal) were processed by specific Cardio 200 program for volume calculation according to Chapman's biplanar method.

The program divides the ventricle into slices of 2 mm and adds the single slice volumes together according to Simpson's rule. The longer of the two axes is selected and the smaller contour is transformed accordingly. The other methodologic details were the same as described under point 1. The procedure was applied in 32 echocardiographic studies.

3. Tricuspid annular plane systolic excursion (TAPSE)

Employing the video recordings of the right ventricle in the apical 4-chamber view, we measured the distance between the centre of origin of the echocardiographic fan to the junction of the tricuspid valve with the RV lateral wall. The shortening of this distance from end-diastole to end-systole represents the tricuspid annular plane systolic excursion described by Kaul et al. in 1984[6] as a simple and accurate predictor of RV systolic function.

The TAPSE measurement was performed in 31 patient studies. The variability of repeated measurements of RV area and length expressed by variation coefficient was 4 and 7%, respectively.

For statistical evaluation of the results we used paired t-test and linear regression analysis. The values of sensitivity, specificity, positive and negative prediction and overall accuracy were calculated according to previously described formulas.[14]

Results

Table I presents the mean values of RV end-diastolic (EDV), end-systolic (ESV) and stroke volume (SV) together with derived ejection fraction (EF) estimated from images of both applied techniques - RV angiography and echocardiographic area-length method. While there were no significant differences between the means of end-systolic volume and ejection fraction, a slight but systematic underestimation of end-diastolic and stroke volumes by echocardiography was proved by paired t-test.

The linear regression analysis exhibits the close correlation of right ventricular EDV and ESV derived from echocardiography with the same variables obtained from angiography (Fig. 2). The correlation coefficients exceed 0.8 and the devia-

Table I. The RV volumes and ejection fraction derived from angiography (all volumes are expressed as indexes per 1 m^2 of body surface area).

	EDVI	ESVI	SVI	EF
Angio	106.11±32.52	46.98±23.70	59.16±15.50	0.57±0.10
Echo	99.43±39.45	47.41±25.67	53.68±19.73	0.56±0.10
	*	+	**	+

* $p<0.05$; ** $p<0.01$; + NS

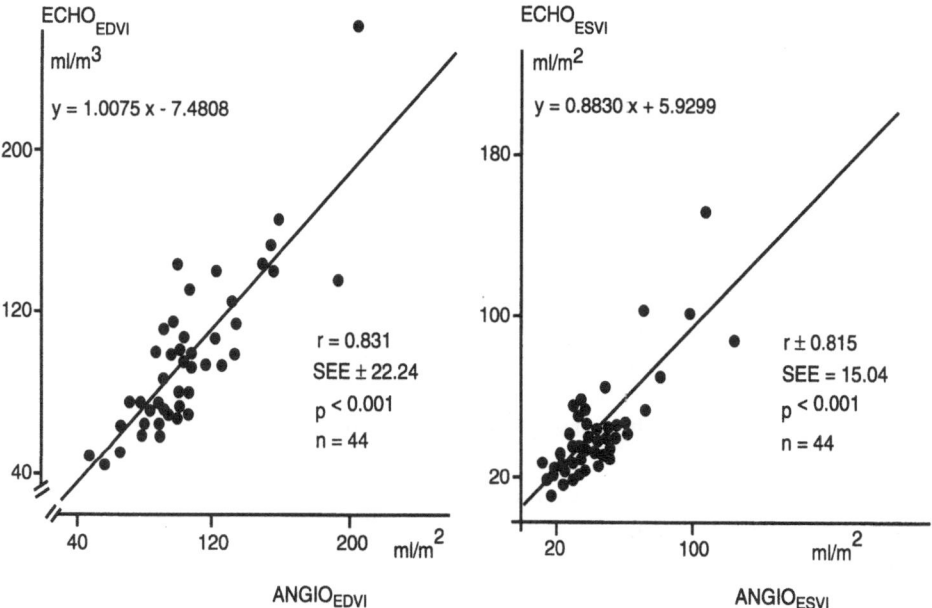

Fig. 2. The correlation of RV end-diastolic and end-systolic volumes calculated from echocardiographic and angiographic images (abbreviations:see text, all volumes are expressed as indexes per 1 m^2 of body surface area).

tion of regression lines from identity seems negligible. The correlation of SV and EF found is also favourable (Fig. 3).

The slight deviation of the regression line in EF is mainly caused by underestimated values of EDV by echocardiography.

On the other hand, applying Simpson's rule for RV volume and function estimation from two orthogonal echo-planes defined above led to discouraging results. The values of parameters investigated by echocardiography were:

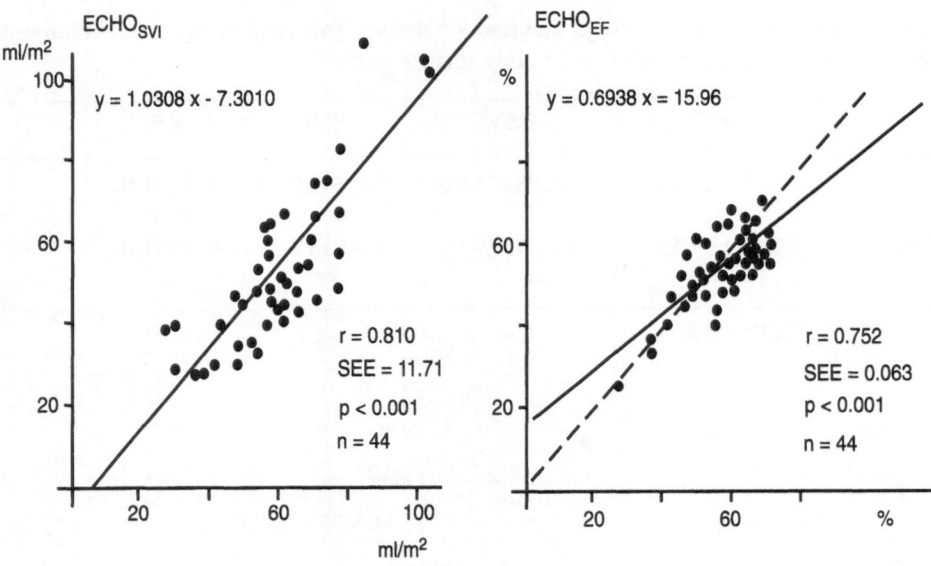

Fig. 3. The correlation of derived variables - stroke volume (SV) and ejection fraction (EF).

$EDV=49,3\pm24,7$ ml/m^2, $ESV=27,3\pm20,2$ ml/m^2, $SV=22,3\pm7,0$ ml/m^2, $EF=0.48\pm0.11$. The same values derived from cine-angiography were as follows: $EDV=104.6\pm35.7$ ml/m^2, $ESV=46.2\pm26.7$ ml/m^2, $SV=58.7\pm16.0$ ml/m^2, $EF=0,58\pm0,11$. Echocardiography exhibited an apparent underestimation of all RV volumes, differing from angiography on the same level of statistical significance ($p<0,001$, paired t-test). The correlations between individual variables were loose (Tab. II).

The mean of tricuspid annular plane systolic excursion (TAPSE) in 31 patient studies was 1.46 ± 0.53 cm. The correlation of TAPSE with EF determined by angiography was poor and statistically insignificant ($r=0.288$; $SEE=0.514$; $p>0.1$).

Trying to fix the most practical value of the echocardiographic area-length method in RV function evaluation, we checked this approach in differentiating those subjects with decreased angiographic EF from those with normal values.

Angiographic values of EF equal to or exceeding 0.60 are considered normal in our catheterization department. Because of the slight underestimation of higher EF by echocardiography (see the slope of the regression line in Fig. 3), the value of 0.55 was accepted as borderline for this technique.

Using the described approach we were able to recognize correctly 68% of RV failure detected by angiography, with 82% specificity and satisfactory values of prediction and overall accuracy (Tab. III).

Studying the possible influence of tricuspid regurgitation (TR) on RV ejection fraction, we correlated the echocardiographic and angiographic EF with the mean

Table II. The correlations of echocardiographic volumes and ejection fraction with angiographic data (Simpson's rule was applied in echocardiographic evaluation)

		$Angio_{RV}$ (Ferlinz)			
		EDVI	ESVI	SVI	EF
2D-Echo (Simpson)	r	* 0.512	** 0.636	+ 0.319	** 0.621
	SEE	21.50	15.88	6.77	0.089
	(n = 32)				

* p<0.01; ** p<0.001; + NS

Table III. Detection of RV dysfunction: $EF_{ECHO} < 0.55$

Sensitivity	0.68	+predictive value	0.79
Specificity	0.82	-predictive value	0.72
Overall accuracy	0.75		

pulmonary artery pressure (PAP) measured directly at catheterization. While a significant correlation was proved in patients without TR (Fig. 4) the relation between echocardiographic and angiographic EF and PAP in the presence of any degree of TR was insignificant (r = 0.283 and 0.194, respectively; n.s.).

Discussion

As it has been demonstrated previously in chronic lung diseases, the long-term survival is obviously related to presence or absence of the signs of right ventricular failure.[10,13] Therefore, we can assume, the data concerning the right ventricular ejection fraction as a measure of its systolic function represent an important indicator in clinical evaluation of individual patients.

Right heart catheterization together with RV angiography remain the reference methods in such cases. However, in a long-term follow-up of the natural course and the effect of treatment of any particular disease, the appropriate non-invasive RV function assessment should be appreciated.

Concerning this point, radionuclide angiography has gained an accepted position in cardiological research and sometimes also in daily practice. Nevertheless, the expensive equipment prevents its routine use in many established hospitals. In

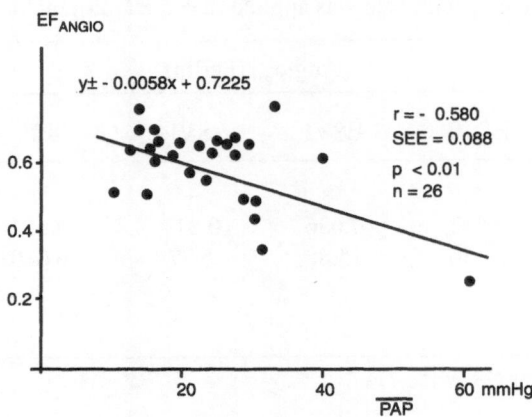

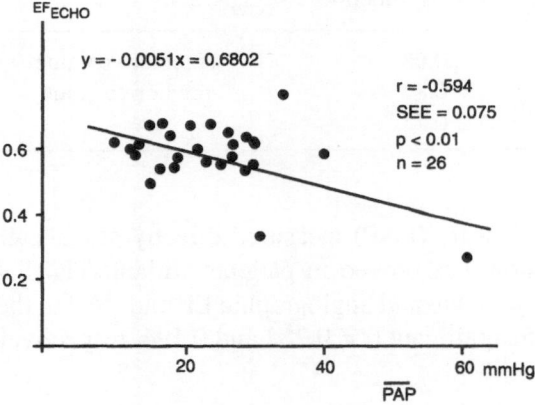

Fig. 4. The correlation of echocardiographic and angiographic ejection fraction (EF) with mean pulmonary artery pressure (PAP) in patients without tricuspid insufficiency (TI-).

contrast, echocardiography, as clinically widespread a diagnostic method, offers an alternative and easily accessible approach to noninvasive evaluation of RV function. This fact represented the basic rationale for initiating our study.

During recent years, some reasonable correlations between 2D echocardiographic measurements of right ventricular volumes and their angiographic (contrast or radionuclide) assessment have been described; nevertheless, no approach has achieved widespread use and evaluation of the right ventricle has remained primarily qualitative.

Having been attracted by some encouraging reports, we decided to test several recently introduced echocardiographic techniques of RV volume and/or function evaluation and compare them with findings of RV angiography in order to choose the best one for current clinical use. In agreement with two model studies on RV cast volumes,[8,4] the area-length method, calculating the volume of the half-cylindrical, half-conical RV, has appeared accurate enough also in human study. Actually, the correlation coefficients of echo- and angio-estimated RV volumes are slightly lower compared with their high value in RV cast measurements (0.95 - 0.98), but there are some apparent factors responsible for the differences between the two techniques:

1. the measurements were performed separately (within a 7 day interval) and some day-to-day subclinical changes in patient haemodynamic conditions could not be ruled out, as have been demonstrated for the left ventricular dimensions and ejection fraction;[9]
2. the technique of echocardiographic measurement in humans is completely different, more tedious and image quality is not so good as in the experimental setting;
3. finally, the angiographic RV volumes evaluation was performed from single-plane RV angiography instead of the biplane one employed in the original study;[4] this suboptimal standard was due to the available equipment.

The next limiting factor might be angiography alone, as a "gold standard" for echocardiography. A markedly irregular RV cavity shape has led to different and even more sophisticated geometrical approximations, whose accuracy in some individual cases would be questionable.

In spite of the above-mentioned factors, adversely influencing our results, the correlations found between RV volumes and ejection fraction were better than expected and in general, suitable for clinical application. The underestimation of higher ejection fractions was due to the incorrect end-diastolic RV area, caused most probably by RV trabeculation interfering with the actual RV cavity inner surface delineation. The individual observer's experience of RV cavity area tracing may also play an important role.

Employing Simpson's rule for RV volume and function evaluation from two orthogonal planes used in this study yielded rather discouraging results. A marked underestimation of echo-calculated RV end-diastolic and end-systolic volumes invalidated the assessment of function as well. Our results seem contrary to those of Watanabe's original study,[16] but the difference in echo-projections employed can clearly explain this discordance. While two apical echo-planes exhibit an obviously comparable area,[16] according to our experience, the subcostal RV outflow tract projection area is often smaller than the apical 4-chamber one. However, the original approach is open to criticism for neglecting the RV infundibulum as a constant part of the right ventricular body. We believe, the ideal echocardiographic technique must calculate with both the inflow and outflow part of the right ventricle.

The results of our study are also not able to confirm the extremely favourable findings of Kaul et al.[6] evaluating the tricuspid annular plane systolic excursion as an accurate predictor of RV ejection function. The correlation found with angiographic ejection fraction was much poorer than the original one (0.29 vs. 0.92) and its diagnostic power weaker. Using 15 mm of TAPSE as borderline value between normal and depressed RV function,[6] the observed sensitivity remained reasonable (0,68), but specificity was too low (0.38). From this point of view, this variable seems useless in practice. Seemingly, there are two reasons for our apparently negative results:

1. the possible inaccuracy in the technique of tricuspid annular movement estimation, due to the varying echocardiographic image quality;
2. the exclusion of the RV outflow tract from functional assessment.

The application of 2D echocardiography in RV failure detection remains still partially unresolved. Using the described echocardiographic area-length method and RV angiography as a "gold standard" we were able to recognize correctly slightly more than 2/3 of angio-documented RV dysfunctions. Our data indicate that the borderline values in individual cases are to be interpreted very carefully.

The other point of our study was to provide evidence that tricuspid regurgitation interferes significantly with the RV ejection fraction-pulmonary artery pressure relation. In agreement with a similar recent study,[11] we believe that at a given pulmonary artery pressure, tricuspid regurgitation enhances the RV ejection fraction. The ejection in the presence of tricuspid insufficiency includes both the forward and regurgitant stroke volume, clearly overestimating the resulting ejection fraction.

Consequently, the EF in such cases need not necessarily decline even in RV failure and the changes after successful treatment may remain hidden. Therefore, an ejection fraction as a measure of RV systolic function is of limited value in the presence of any degree of tricuspid regurgitation.

Conclusion

Of the three recently described approaches to RV volume and function assessment, only echocardiographic area-length method yielded satisfactory results in comparison with RV angiography in our clinical setting, providing a good quality echo-image at least.

The echocardiographic diagnosis of RV failure remains limited and great care is recommended in evaluation of borderline EF values. The presence of tricuspid regurgitation leads to the overestimation of the actual EF. The standardization of the technique and further extensive clinical studies are undoubtedly needed.

References

1. Bommer W., Weinert L., Neumann A., Heff J., Mason D.T., DeMaria A.: Determination of right atrial and right ventricular size by two-dimensional echocardiography. Circulation 1979; 60,1:91-100
2. Ferlinz J.: Angiographic assessment of right ventricular volumes and ejection fraction. Cath. Cardiovasc. Diagnosis 1976; 2:5
3. Ferlinz J.: Measurements of right ventricular volumes in man from single plane cineangiograms. Am. Heart J. 1977; 94,1:87-90
4. Gibson T.C., Miller S.W., Aretz T., Hardin N.J., Weyman A.E.: Method for estimating right ventricular volume by planes applicable to cross-sectional echocardiography: Correlation with angiographic formulas. Am. J. Cardiol. 1985; 55:1584-1588
5. Hiraishi S., DiSessa T.G., Jarmakani J.M., Nanakishi T., Isabel-Jones J.B., Friedman W.F.: Two-dimensional echocardiographic assessment of right ventricular volume in children with congenital heart disease. Am. J. Cardiol. 1982; 50:1368-1375
6. Kaul S., Tei Ch., Hopkins J.M., Shah P.M.: Assessment of right ventricular function using two-dimensional echocardiography. Am. Heart J. 1984; 107,3:526-531
7. Konstam M.A., Pandian N.: Assessment of right ventricular function. In: Konstam M.A., Isner J.M. (Eds) *The right ventricle*. Amsterdam, Kluwer Acad. Publ. 1988; 1-15
8. Levine R.A., Gibson T.C., Aretz T., Gillam L.D., Guyer D.E., King M.E., Weyman A.E.: Echocardiographic measurement of right ventricular volume. Circulation 1984; 69,3:497-505
9. McAnulty J.H., Kremkau E.L., Rosh J., Rahimtoola S.H.: Spontaneous changes in left ventricular function between sequential studies. Am. J. Cardiol. 1974; 34:23-28
10. Mitchell R.S., Weeb N.C., Filley G.F.: Chronic obstructive bronchopulmonary disease III. Factors influencing prognosis. Am. Rev. Resp. Dis. 1964; 89:878-896
11. Morrison D.A., Owit T., Hammermeister K.E.: Functional tricuspid regurgitation and right ventricular dysfunction in pulmonary hypertension. Am. J. Cardiol. 1988; 62,1:108-112
12. Ninomiya K., Duncan W.J., Cook D.H., Olley P.M., Rowe R.D.: Right ventricular ejection fraction and volumes after Mustard repair: Correlation of two dimensional echocardiograms and cineangiograms. Am. J. Cardiol. 1981; 48:317-324
13. Ourednik A., Jezek V., Bakova O.: Pronostic de l'hypertension pulmonaire chez les sujects atteints de bronchite chronique. Bull. Physiopath. Resp. 1968; 4:213-224
14. Remington R.D., Schork M.A.: Statistics with applications to the biological and health sciences. New York, Prentice-Hall 1985
15. Starling M.R., Crawford M.H., Sorensen S.G., O'Rourke R.A.: A new two-dimensional echocardiographic technique for evaluating right ventricular size and performance in patients with obstructive lung disease. Circulation 1982; 66,3:612-620
16. Watanabe T., Katsume, Matsukubo H., Furukawa K., Ijibhi H.: Estimation of right ventricular volume with two dimensional echocardiography. Am. J. Cardiol. 1982; 49:1946-1953

13. Right Ventricular Ejection Fraction and Volumes at Rest and During Low Load Exercise in Chronic Lung Disease Patients With and Without Past Right Heart Failure

F. SCHRIJEN[1], J. REDONDO[2], A. HENRIQUEZ[2], J.M. POLU[2]

1. INSERM, Unit 14, Vandoeuvre, Nancy, France
2. CHU Brabois, Vandoeuvre, Nancy, France

Introduction

During the clinical course of chronic lung disease, acute exacerbations due to pulmonary infection are often observed. These may lead to cardiorespiratory failure, with clinical and haemodynamic signs of right heart failure.[1] When the patients recover from the acute episode, blood gases and pulmonary haemodynamics usually return close to their values in stable clinical condition: the evolution of pulmonary artery pressure is less than 1 mmHg per year when patients are studied in stable condition.[2,3]

Right ventricular function seems to be restored as the clinical signs of right heart failure subside, but it is known from experimental studies that when congestive heart failure occurred in the course of right ventricular hypertrophy by pressure overload, the relief of the pressure overload did not allow total recovery of the contractile properties of the myocardium in cats.[4]

One of the best ways to assess ventricular contractile properties at the present stage of knowledge seems to be to consider the ventricular end-systolic pressure/volume relationship[5], and especially its slope.[6]

But the right ventricular volume cannot be easily estimated by imaging procedures because of its peculiar shape. It is possible, however, to derive right ventricular volume from stroke volume and ejection fraction. Using a fast-response thermistor catheter, these variables can be measured together with vascular pressures.

We used this technique in patients with chronic lung disease, with or without a past history of right heart failure.

Methods

Patients

The study was performed in 36 patients with chronic lung disease, in a stable clinical condition. Mean age was 54.5 ± 1.6 (SEM) years. Diagnosis included chronic bronchitis (n=22), with radiological signs of lung distension in 13 cases, pneumoconiosis (n=4), tuberculosis sequelae (n=3), bronchiectasis (n=3), and lung fibrosis (n= 4). The patients were divided according to the presence or absence of right heart failure (RHF) episodes in the course of their disease: 25 patients had no positive history (group 1, without past RHF), and 11 patients had a positive history of RHF (group 2, with past RHF). The patients with chronic bronchitis and those with other diseases were evenly distributed in the two groups, except the 4 patients with pneumoconiosis, who were all in group 1 as none of them had experienced right heart failure.

Protocol

One the day before the procedure, the patients were taken into the catheterization laboratory for a training session: the aim of this session was to get them familiar with the equipment and to determine their ability to exercise. Ventilation, oxygen consumption and CO_2 output were measured with a closed circuit spirometer (Metabograph, Lausanne) to which the subjects were connected via an air-tight facial mask. Only those patients who were able to perform either 40 or 20 W for ten minutes and in whom ventilation did not increase during the last five minutes entered the protocol, since the measurements needed to be made under stable conditions at rest as well as during exercise.

After this training session the patients gave informed consent to the haemodynamic investigation.

Right heart catheterization was performed in the morning, without premedication. The patients were fasting; they were in the supine position for the whole procedure. During exercise however the feet were slightly raised to reach the pedals of the ergometer. Because of the blood volume shift likely to occur in this position[7], we measured right ventricular volume before exercise.

The periods of measurements were thus as follows: rest supine (RS), rest with legs raised (LR), first exercise (loadless pedalling, 0 W, or 20 W, E_1) and second exercise (20 or 40 W, E_2).

Techniques

A Swan-Ganz thermodilution catheter (7.5 F) was advanced via an arm vein under ECG and fluoroscopic monitoring until its tip was in the pulmonary artery. The pressure from the proximal lumen was then monitored in order to place the lumen in the right atrium, close to the tricuspid valve. To measure ejection fraction

10 ml saline were injected rapidly into the right atrium. During the injection the temperature of the injectate was measured between the syringe and the catheter. It ranged from 7 to 14°C. The Swan-Ganz catheter was also used to measure vascular pressures. A plastic needle was inserted into the contralateral brachial artery for blood sampling and pressure measurements.

For each period, the measurements included blood gases, ventilatory and haemodynamic variables. Oxygen saturation was measured with a haemoxymeter (OSM 2, Radiometer, Copenhagen), pH, oxygen and CO_2 partial pressure with ABL (Radiometer), ventilation and oxygen consumption were computed every minute with the Metabograph, a closed circuit spirometer to which the patient was connected via a facial mask, vascular pressures were measured with Thomson-Telco manometers and recorded by a photographic procedure. The reference level for atmospheric pressure was midway between the sternal notch and the table plane. The zero pressure was recorded after each measurement. A static calibration was performed after each study with a mercury manometer.

Derived variables

Pulmonary vascular resistance (PVR, $dyn.s.cm^{-5}$) was computed as $80 (\overline{P}pa - Pw)$ where mean pulmonary artery pressure ($\overline{P}pa$) and mean wedge pressure ($\overline{P}w$) were expressed in mmHg, and cardiac output in l/min. Right ventricular end-diastolic volume (RVEDV,ml) was computed as stroke volume (SV)/RVEF, and right ventricular end-systolic volume (RVESV, ml) as RVEDV - SV.

Statistical analysis

The results are expressed as mean ± SEM. To compare mean values from groups of patients the standard t-test was used, and a paired t-test was used to compare different periods in the same patients. Relationships between variables were studied by regression analysis and correlation coefficient.[8]

Results

Lung function variables and blood gases are shown in Table I. Both groups showed airways obstruction, which was more severe in group 2 (positive history of RHF), but the difference between groups was significant for VC and FEV_1 (% predicted) only. $PaCO_2$ was close to the upper limit of normal in group 2, and PaO_2 was close to the upper limit of normal in group 2, and PaO_2 was lower on average in group 1, but the difference was not significant.

Haemodynamic data are shown in Table II. At rest supine, only PVR was statistically more elevated in group 2. This difference became more significant with legs raised, and pulmonary artery pressure and wedge pressure became also significantly higher in group 2.

Table I. Lung function and blood gases in patients with chronic lung disease divided according to their past history of right heart failure (RHF)

Past RHF:	without	with	p
n:	25	11	
VC (%pred)	84±5	65±5	<0.01
FEV_1 (%pred)	61±6	39±3	<0.01
FEV_1/VC (%)	56±3	50±5	
RV/TLC (%)	47±3	58±4	
TLC (%pred)	97±3	101±6	
$PaCO_2$ (mmHg)	39.6±1.3	43.8±1.0	<0.05
PaO_2 (mmHg)	63±3	57±3	

Mean±SEM; %pred, values as a percentage of predicted valves[9]

Ejection fraction was close to the lower limit of normal in group 1 and it increased with exercise, whereas in group 2 it was lower and did not change with exercise. The difference between the groups however was significant for E_1 only. Although the right ventricular volumes were not statistically different, they tended to be lower in group 1, particularly during exercise.

The relation between end-diastolic pressure and end-diastolic pressure in the right ventricle, is shown in figure 1, for the four periods of measurements. The changes from rest supine (R) to rest with legs raised (LR) were parallel in the two groups, however the first exercise level (E_1) produced a larger volume and pressure increase, with a slope more towards the volume axis in group 2; from E_1 to E_2, there was almost no change in group 1, but in group 2 a further increase in volume and in pressure was observed, and the slope became more vertical.

The right ventricular end-systolic pressure/volume relation is shown in figure 2. The difference between the patients without and with a past history of RHF is more obvious than for the end-diastolic relation: right ventricular end-systolic volume hardly changed in group 1, but both pressure and volume increased with exercise in group 2, showing a decreased contractility despite the sympathetic stimulation due to exercise.

Considering the changes in stroke volume with end-diastolic volume as an indicator of preload (Fig. 3), the rest supine to legs raised slope was similar in groups 1 and 2, but from rest to exercise the changes were opposite: in group 1 the slope increased, presumably due to the increase in sympathetic tone during exercise, but this was ineffective in group 2, where the slope decreased with exercise.

Table II. Haemodynamic values at rest supine (R) and with the legs raised (LR), and during two stages of low load exercise (E_1 and E_2).

Past RHF	without				with			
	R	LR	E_1	E_2	R	LR	E_1	E_2
RVEDP	3.6	5.2	6.0	6.1	2.9	4.5	6.1	7.7
(mmHg)	0.5	0.6	0.6	0.7	0.5	0.9	1.0	1.0
$\overline{\text{PAP}}$	20.8	24.0	31.0	34.0	25.7	30.7[*]	40.5[*]	47.0[**]
(mmHg)	1.3	1.4	2.0	2.0	2.2	2.3	2.9	3.4
$\overline{\text{Pw}}$	8.2	10.9	13.8	14.8	5.6	7.5[*]	11.2	12.6
(mmHg)	0.7	0.8	1.0	1.4	1.1	1.4	2.2	2.5
$\overline{\text{Pa}}$	105	114	118	120	102	110	117	124
(mmHg)	4	4	4	4	5	6	7	8
$\dot{Q}$	5.4	5.9	7.6	9.1	5.6	5.9	7.8	9.3
(l/min)	0.2	0.2	0.3	0.4	0.3	0.3	0.4	0.5
HR	76.7	77.7	90.8	99.0	81.1	82.3	96.5	109.3[*]
(b/min)	2.6	2.4	2.3	2.5	3.2	3.7	4.2	4.2
SV	74	78	85	94	70	74	83	86
(ml)	3	4	4	5	5	5	6	6
PVR	191	187	195	181	305[*]	327[**]	319[*]	311[*]
(dyn.s.cm⁻⁵)	20	19	22	20	50	45	45	51
RVEF	0.38	0.38	0.41	0.44	0.34	0.35	0.34[*]	0.36
	0.02	0.02	0.02	0.02	0.02	0.03	0.03	0.03
RVEDV	202	211	219	223	213	221	256	263
(ml)	10	11	11	13	12	14	21	28
RVESV	128	133	133	129	143	147	174	175
(ml)	10	10	11	11	12	16	20	29

Mean and standard error.
RHF: right heart failure; RVEDP: right ventricular end-diastolic pressure; $\overline{\text{PAP}}$: mean pulmonary artery pressure; $\overline{\text{Pw}}$: mean wedge pressure; $\overline{\text{Pa}}$: mean systemic arterial pressure; $\dot{Q}$: cardiac output; PVR: pulmonary vascular resistance; RVEF, right ventricular ejection fraction; RVEDV: right ventricular end-diastolic volume; RVESV: right ventricular end-systolic volume. Significance of the differences between groups: $*p<0.05$, $**p<0.01$.

The patients in group 1 differed from those in group 2 in their past history of right heart failure. But PVR was significantly higher in group 2, and this increased afterload could in itself be the cause of the differences observed as far as right

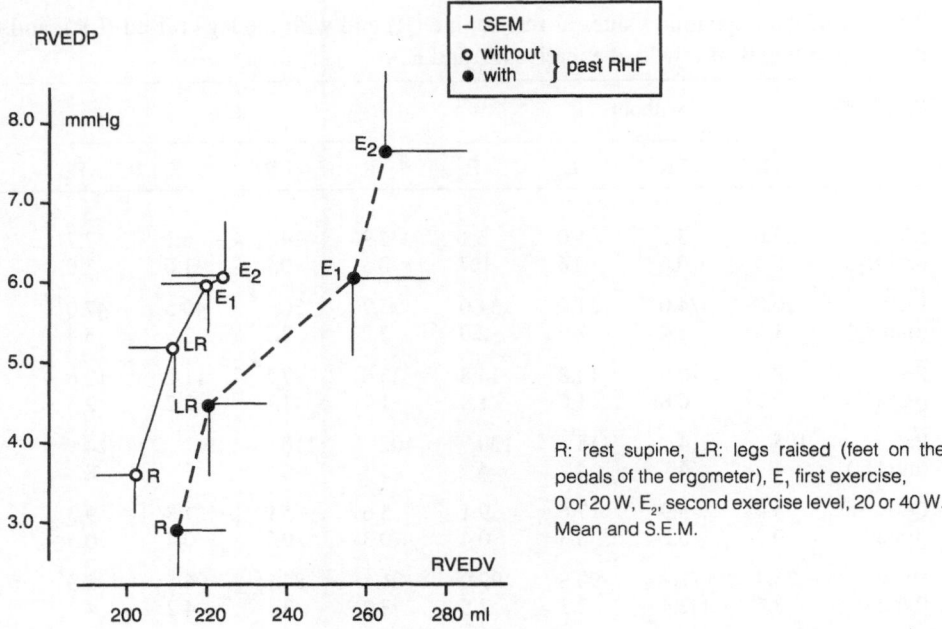

Fig. 1. Relationship between right ventricular end-diastolic pressure (RVEDP) and right ventricular end-diastolic volume (RVEDV) in two groups of subjects with chronic lung disease.

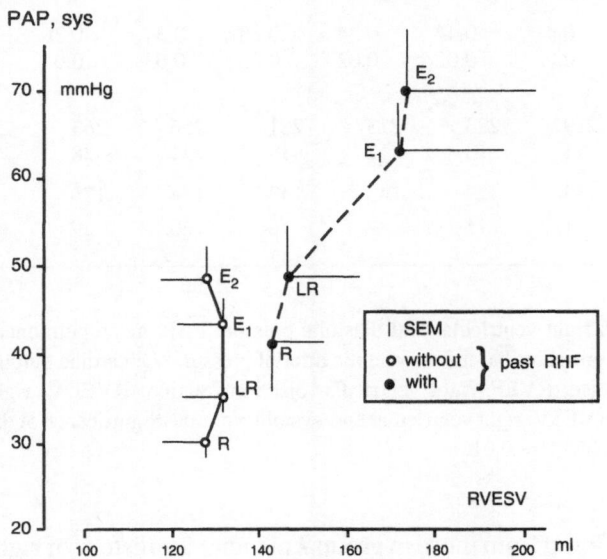

Fig. 2. Relationship between pulmonary arterial systolic pressure (PAP, sys) and right ventricular end-systolic volume (RVESV). For symbols, see Fig. 1.

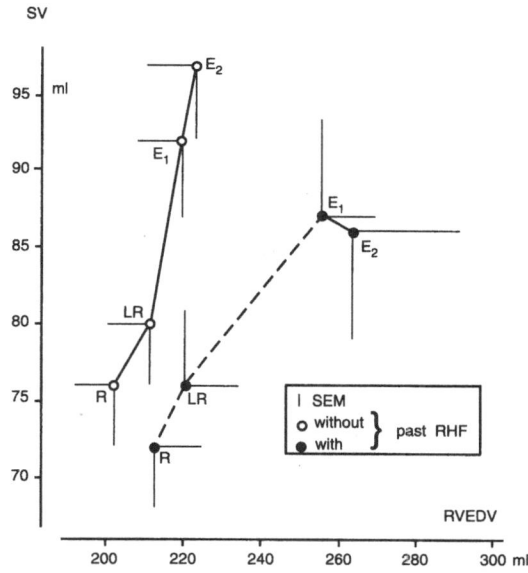

Fig. 3. Changes in stroke volume (SV) related to right ventricular end-diastolic volume (RVEDV). For symbols, see Fig. 1.

ventricular function was concerned. For this reason we tried to choose in group 1 patients who matched those from group 2 for $PaCO_2$, PaO_2 and PVR.

This was possible for 9 patients only, from group 1 (called group 1M) and group 2 (group 2M). As expected, RVEF was lower in group 1M than in group 1 at rest supine (0.31 ± 0.02) and with legs raised (0.35 ± 0.04), but it increased normally with exercise: 0.37 ± 0.04 during E_1 and 0.43 ± 0.04 during E_2. It was similar at rest in group 2M: 0.33 ± 0.03 supine, 0.35 ± 0.04 with legs raised, but remained unchanged with exercise: 0.34 ± 0.03 during E_1 and 0.34 ± 0.04 during E_2.

The difference in the systolic pressure/volume relation for the right ventricle was even more striking when the matched groups were considered (Fig. 4): there was no difference at rest, but exercise produced an increase in right ventricular end-systolic volume in the group with a positive history of RHF (2M), while RVESV decreased in the group without past RHF (1M).

The difference in RVESV change from LR to E_2 was significant ($p < 0.05$). A significant difference ($p < 0.05$) was also observed for the change in right ventricular end-diastolic volume from LR to E_2.

The changes in stroke volume and in RVEDV are shown in figure 5. In group 1M the right ventricular function is stimulated with exercise, especially as the second level, whereas in group 2M it is depressed, with an increase in RVEDV without change in stroke volume, from E_1 to E_2.

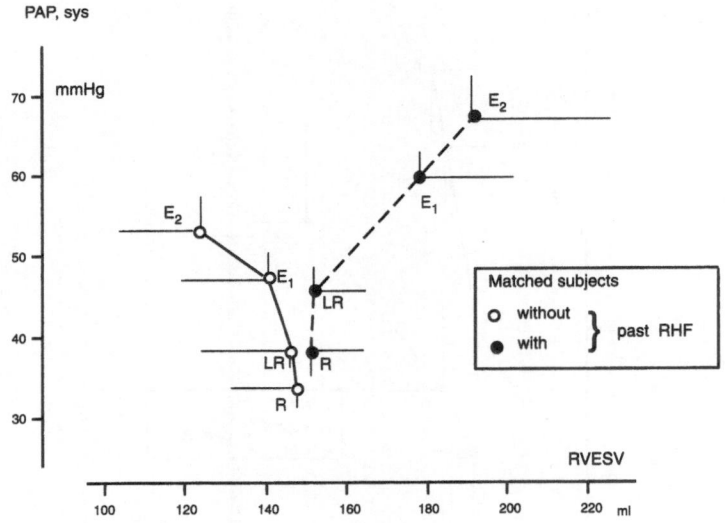

Fig. 4. Pulmonary arterial systolic pressure (PAP, sys) and right ventricular end-systolic volume (RVESV) changes from rest to exercise. (o): 9 patients without past history of RHF, matched for $PaCO_2$, PaO_2 and RVP with 9 patients with a positive history of RHF (●). For symbols, see Fig. 1.

Discussion

Measuring right ventricular ejection fraction together with the more classical variables in the pulmonary circulation allows a better evaluation in patients with chronic lung disease, since it makes it possible the study of end-systolic and end-diastolic pressure/volume relationships for the right ventricle. We measured the right ventricular pressure after the atrial contraction as end-diastolic pressure, and end-systolic pressure was taken as the peak pressure on the pulmonary arterial pressure curve, which is probably closer to the end-systolic pressure than that of the dicrotic notch, because of the uncertainty about the end of ejection in the right ventricle.[10]

Our results showed a lower RVEF at rest in the patients with than in the patients without a positive history of RHF. Because RVEF is afterload dependent[11], we matched patients for PVR, and this time RVEF at rest was similar in both groups. But the same changes with exercise were still observed, i.e., an increase in RVEF in group 1M, without past episodes of RHF, and no change in group 2M, with a positive history of RHF. In a previous work[12] we observed that RVEF at rest was related to lung function assessed by spirometry and blood gases. This may be due to the fact that the patients were studied away from acute episodes. The present study shows that the RVEF changes occurring during exercise depend on the presence of previous RHF episodes. Since RVEF is influenced by preload, afterload and contractility, we studied pressure-volume relations to try to isolate these factors. We used a passive increase in venous return (from supine to legs raised) and an active increase in cardiac output, which is accompanied by a shift in autonomous nervous activity towards a higher sympathetic tone. For this reason the points representing rest and exercise values cannot be considered as being on the same cardiac function curve.[13]

Nevertheless, the comparison between our patients groups shows that with exercise the pressure-volume relation improved in group 1 and deteriorated in group 2. Also the relation between stroke volume and RVEDV was impaired with the second level of exercise in group 2 and especially in group 2M, where end-diastolic volume continued to increased without change in stroke volume (Fig. 5).

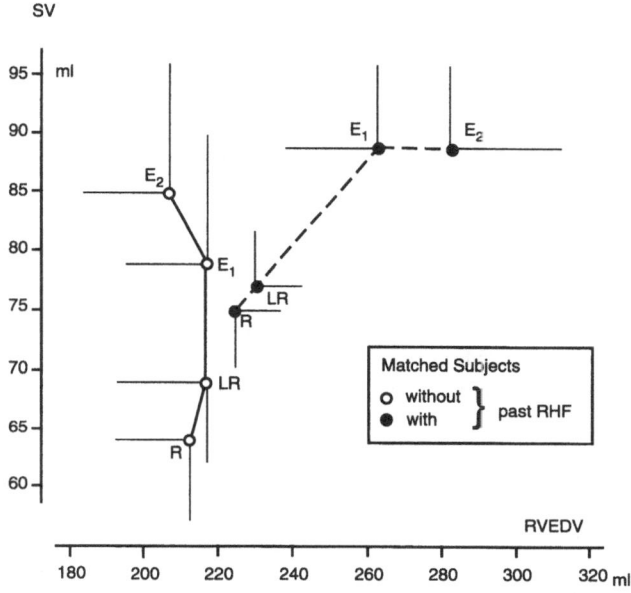

Fig. 5. Relationship between stroke volume (SV) and right ventricular end-diastolic volume (RVEDV) at rest and during exercise, in two groups of nine patients matched for $PaCO_2$, PaO_2 and RVP. (○): no past history of RHF, (●): positive history of RHF. For symbols, see Fig. 1.

Experimental work has shown that after reversal of right ventricular pressure overload hypertrophy, some structural changes remain, with an increased proportion of collagenous proteins.[14]

In our patients with a positive history of RHF it also seems that there are some permanent changes which lead to a worsening of the right ventricular pressure-volume relations.

164

Even though lung function seems similar to that in patients who never experienced RHF, their exercise capacity is more limited with respect to right ventricular function.

In conclusion, the history of RHF episodes is important in assessing the right ventricular function in patients with chronic lung disease.

Acknowledgements: The Authors wish to thank F. Poincelot and F. Harmand for tecnical assistance.

References

1. Lockhart A., Tsareva M., Schrijen F., Sadoul P.: Etudes hémodynamiques des décompensations respiratoires aiguës des bronchopneumopathies chroniques. Bull. Physiopath. Resp. 1967; 3:645-667
2. Schrijen F., Uffholtz H., Polu J.M., Poincelot F.: Pulmonary and systemic hemodynamic evolution in chronic bronchitis. Am. Rev. Resp. Dis. 1978; 117:25-31
3. Weitzenblum E., Loiseau A., Hirth C., Mirhom R., Rasaholinjanahary J.: Course of pulmonary haemodynamics in patients with chronic obstructive pulmonary disease. Chest 1979; 75:656-62
4. Coulton R.L., Yazdanfar S., Rubio E., Bove A.A., Lemole G.M., Spann J.F.: Recuperative potential of cardiac muscle following relief of pressure overload hypertrophy and right ventricular failure in the cat. Circulation Res. 1977; 40:41-9
5. Grossman W., Braunwald E., Mann T., McLaurin L.P., Green L.H.: Contractile state of the left ventricle in man as evaluated from end-systolic pressure-volume relations. Circulation 1977; 56:845-52
6. Sagawa K.: The end-systolic pressure-volume relation of the ventricle: definition, modifications and clinical use. Circulation 1981; 63:1223-7
7. Schrijen F., Urtiaga B.: Pulmonary blood volume in chronic lung disease; changes with legs raised and during exercise. Chest, 1982; 81:544-9
8. Snedecor G.W., Cochran W.G.: *Statistical methods.* Ames, Iowa: State University press, 1967
9. Quanjer P., Dalhuijsen A., van Zomeren B.C.: Summary equations of reference values. Bull. Eur. Physiopath. Resp. 1983; 19 suppl. 5:45-51
10. Brown K.A., Ditchey R.V.: Human right ventricular end-systolic pressure-volume relation defined by maximal elastance. Circulation 1988; 78:81-91
11. Morrisson D., Goldman S., Wright A.L., Henry R., Sorenson S., Caldwell J., Ritchie J.: The effect of pulmonary hypertension on systolic function of the right ventricle. Chest 1983; 84:250-7
12. Schrijen F., Redondo J., Henriquez A., De Vito A., Polu J.M.: Right ventricular ejection fraction at rest during two stages of low-load exercise in patients with chronic lung disease. Eur. Heart J. 1988; 9 suppl 1, 356
13. Guyton A.C., Jones C.E., Coleman T.G.: *Circulatory physiology: cardiac output and its regulation.* Philadelphia, Saunders Company 1973
14. Ostadal B., Pelouch V., Kolar F., Prochazka J., Cihak R., Widimsky J.: *Experimental right ventricular hypertrophy.* Pulmonary Circulation V proceedings, Prague 1989; 108

14. Holter Findings in Patients Dying from Chronic Cor Pulmonale

J. DOLENSKY[1], J. WIDIMSKY[2], J. HAMMER[3], K. KROFTA[1]

1. Department of Tuberculosis and Respiratory Diseases, Thomayer's Teaching Hospital, Prague, Czechoslovakia
2. Institute of Physiology, Czechoslovak Academy of Sciences, Postgraduate Medical School, Prague, Czechoslovakia
3. Department of Medicine, Institute for Clinical and Experimental Medicine, Prague, Czechoslovakia

Introduction

The incidence of cardiac dysrhythmias in patients with cor pulmonale is high, as suggested by reports published in various countries. Despite this, the prognostic value of cardiac dysrhythmias in these patients has not been defined yet in view of the problems involved.

The aim of our study was to compare the incidence of cardiac dysrhythmias in a group of living subjects and another one made up of patients who had died from cor pulmonale.

The diagnosis of chronic cor pulmonale was established by clinical examination, electrocardiography, x-ray, and by post mortem examination in dead patients.

Patients and Methods

In the first part of the study, a group of 60 patients was subjected to 24-hour Holter monitoring (Table I) using a Del Mar Avionics system. Their basic data are given in Table II. It is evident from the table that 3/4 of the group were men with a mean age of 63 years. They were mostly patients with obstructive pulmonary disease, as shown by the next table (Table III).

All patients had respiratory failure, and a number of them also signs of right-heart cardiac failure. To assess the dysrhythmias, a modified Lown scale, proposed in the study by Klieger et al.,[4] was employed (Table IV). Our definition of severe dysrhythmia was grade 3 or more on the scale.

Table I. Dysrhythmia in cor pulmonale. Examination by Holter electrocardiography

Type of device	Del Mar avionics
Monitoring period	24 hours (8 a.m. - 8 a.m.) day 6 a.m. - 10 p.m., night 10 p.m. - 6 a.m.
Number of patients	60

Table II. Basic characteristics of patient group

Number	Male	Female	Mean age (range)
60	45(75%)	15(25%)	63 (25-79)

Table III. Patient stratification by diagnosis

COLD	Fibroses	Others (Kyphoscoliosis)
54	4	2

Table IV. Classification of ectopic heart rhythm according to Lown

Atrial arrhytmias: APC (Atrial Premature Contraction)

A0 .... Without APC
A1 .... Unifocal APC
A2 .... Unifocal APC greater than 10/hour
A3 .... Multifocal APC
A4 .... Paired APC
A5 .... Atrial fibrillation
A6 .... Multifocal atrial tachycardia

Ventricular arrhythmias: VPC /Ventricular premature contraction)

V0 .... Without VPC
V1 .... Unifocal VPC
V2 .... Unifocal VPC greater than 10/hour
V3 .... Multifocal VPC
V4 .... Paired VPC
V5 .... Ventricular tachycardia

Results

Results of the examination are given in Table V. Fifty-eight percent of the group showed severe, predominantly supraventricular, dysrhythmias.

In the second part of the study, carried out two years later, the data of Holter monitoring obtained in those patients of our group who had died, were examined. The findings are shown in Table VI.

A total of 10 patients, i.e., 17% died in the meantime. Holter monitoring in most dead patients was performed within one month before death. Basic characteristics of the dead patients are listed in Table VII.

Statistical comparison of the groups of living and dead patients with regard to age, FEV_1 and paO_2 did not reveal significant differences (using the t-test, all were non-significant), and showed both groups are comparable. The basic diagnosis in the overwhelming majority of dead (8 patients) was obstructive bronchopulmonary disease.

Table V. Detection rate of examination: severe dysrhythmias (grade 3 or more by Klieger classification)

Total 35 patients			58%
of these:	atrial	36	60%
	ventricular 11		18%

Table VI. Deaths

Number 10	Follow-up period	Follow-up interval before death
(17%)	2 years	within one month - 7 cases within one year - 3 cases

Table VII. Group of dead patients: characteristics

Number	Male	Female	Age (range)	FEV_1 (%)	paO_2 (kPa)
10	7	3	62 (39-75)	36 (21-76)	7.2 (5.1-9.2)

Table VIII. Group of dead patients. Analysis of memoport.

	Number	%
Positive memoport	10	100
Predominant SVES	10	100
Predominant VES	4	40
Predominantly diurnal	4	40
Predominantly nocturnal	6	60
Presence of ST	6	60
Presence of VT	3	30
Presence of $R_{on}T$	5	50

A thorough analysis of Holter data in dead patients is shown in Table VIII.

This table documents the following observations: all patients (100%) were diagnosed to have severe dysrhythmias, i.e., positive Memoport, with atrial dysrhythmias more frequent than ventricular ones (100 vs. 40%).

Likewise, atrial tachycardias (often polytopic) were more frequent compared with ventricular ones (60 vs. 30%). Half of the dead patients had a positive R on T phenomenon.

Statistical evaluation of the findings obtained in both groups of patients, alive and dead, was performed by Dr. Skibová from the Computer Centre of the Institute for Clinical and Experimental Medicine. The following hypotheses were tested:

1. Is there a difference between the groups of living and dead patients in the incidence of VES? Testing was performed using Pearson's non-parametric test. χ^2 is 5.09.
   Conclusion: there is a difference, at a 5% level of significance, in the incidence of VES between the groups of living and dead patients.

2. Is there a difference between the groups of living and dead patients in the incidence of SVES? χ^2 test value is 8.9, $p < 0.001$.
   Conclusion: a highly statistically significant difference in the incidence of SVES between the groups of living and dead subjects was found.

Discussion

Rhythmias, both atrial and ventricular, are common in cor pulmonale.[4,6] While their frequency is often related to the stage of the underlying disease, the key factor, in our view, is the method of patient selection. Our findings are generally comparable with those reported in the literature. In their study of 25 patients with advanced bronchial obstruction, Klieger and Senior[4] found cardiac dysrhythmias in 84% of patients during 10-hour monitoring (72% had VES and 52% were found to have SVES, mean paO_2 of 60 torr, $paCO_2$ of 45 torr).

Continuous monitoring of the ECG curve reveals a substantially higher incidence of rhythmias compared with standard ECG, and this even when performed repeatedly. However, it should be remembered that various cardiac dysrhythmias may be detected even in fully healthy individuals. Brodsky et al.[1] report, e.g., an incidence of SVES and VES as high as 50% during 24-hour continuous ECG monitoring in 50 healthy individuals.

However, the authors conclude that, despite the high incidence, the total number of dysrhythmias throughout the period of monitoring remains relatively low. In their study, the proportion of patients with a total number of VES over 50/24 hours was as low as 0.5%.

Likewise Clark et al.[2] report that serious cardiac dysrhythmias in healthy individuals are comparably rare. It was for this reason that our definition of significant rhythmias included dysrhythmias such as multifocal SVES or VES, i.e., beginning at grade 3 or more of the Klieger score of ectopic rhythms. Unifocal extrasystoles (even those with a rate exceeding 10/hr) were not considered a serious phenomenon in our evaluation. We are aware the above classification system is a simplification. However, it was the aim of our study to differentiate, in a simple manner, a group of individuals with the less serious dysrhythmias, since most authors fail to do so.

Relationship between diurnal and nocturnal rhythmias

Flick and Block[5] observed the incidence of nocturnal dysrhythmias was twice that of daytime dysrhythmias. In our study, we did not demonstrate a higher incidence of rhythmias during sleep. Another trial, i.e., that by Holford et al.,[6] showed, in a group of 33 hospitalized patients with COLD, diurnal fluctuations in as few as six patients with the highest incidence of cardiac dysrhythmias in the early morning hours. The authors, however, were unable to document diurnal fluctuations in rhythmias in most patients. Moreover, they found that the more frequent SVES were usually associated with VES, but not vice versa.

In our study, we noted a relatively low coincidence of both SVES and VES. Some authors[7,8] also suggest that the incidence of nocturnal hyposaturation in COLD may be associated with the incidence of arrhythmias. However, this is but a hypothesis that must be tested in prospective studies. Moreover, current studies[9] seem to suggest that only the BB type of COLD tends, during arterial blood hyposaturation, to early development of pulmonary hypertension and, consequently, cor pulmonale.

170

The effect of hypoxaemia on the development of cardiac arrhythmias

Most recent studies[10,11] do not demonstrate a significant correlation between arrhythmias and paO_2. Neither did we find a correlation between paO_2 and arrhythmias in our study. The study of Flick, published in 1977, was designed to assess continuous monitoring of the ECG curve in 10 patients. In eight of them, the value of paO_2 was below 40 torr. Nocturnal low-flow oxygenotherapy decreased the incidence of arrhythmias in four patients. However, the reduction in the number of arrhythmias in the group, when seen as a whole, was not statistically significant. Flick recommends monitoring the relationship between SaO_2 and arrhythmias in the future.

To date, our search of the literature has failed to locate a study determining the relationship between the severity of bronchial obstruction and arrhythmias. Our study was designed to compare also the relationship between FEV_1, O_2 and arrhythmias.

As a statistically highly significant correlation was found, we believe the relationship between arrhythmias and blood gas levels must be further studied, and this especially so in patients with severe respiratory insufficiency. The literature fails to offer detailed information regarding the incidence of arrhythmias in this condition. It can be concluded that the mechanism of arrhythmias in COLD remains unclear. The aetiology may be multiple: hypoxaemia, acidosis, digitalis, bronchodilatory therapy and impaired electrolyte balance. The effect of theophylline is reported by the study of Josephson published in 1980.[12] In a group of 41 asthma patients, arrhythmias were found in as little as 20% of patients during an attack. The authors did not find any correlation between dysrhythmias and serum theophylline levels. The role of digitalis was examined in a critical study published by Goren and Denes in 1981.[13] The Authors did not demonstrate a positive correlation between arrhythmias and varied serum digitalis levels determined in 69 patients. Considering the above fact, it is necessary to study these issues in various centres also in the future.

We tried to get a clear-cut answer regarding a possible correlation between cardiac dysrhythmias and SaO_2 values in real time. This important and intriguing problem was suggested in the study of Flick et al. The authors performed 24-hour monitoring of the ECG curve in 10 patients to find a maximum incidence of cardiac dysrhythmias in COLD in the early morning hours (between 3 and 5 a.m.). Apparently sleep is associated with an increased incidence of cardiac dysrhythmias in these patients. Oxygen administration led to a decrease in the incidence of arrhythmias in one fourth of patients.

This shows some patients may benefit from night-time oxygenotherapy. The authors of this paper believe, that, to identify these patients, extensive prospective monitoring trials are necessary. Our study demonstrated that obstructive bronchitis, i.e., BB-type COLD, is associated with significantly more frequent and deeper arterial blood desaturation compared with the emphysema type of COLD.

A similar conclusion was formulated in the study by DeMarco et al.[8] who monitored four patients with the BB type and six patients with the PP type of obstructive pulmonary disease.

The Authors found no difference in total sleep time and incidence of sleep respiratory disturbances. However, patients with prevalent obstructive bronchitis showed more pronounced decreases in SaO_2 during sleep, and lower baseline values of SaO_2 when awaken.

The Authors recommend nocturnal oxygenotherapy in patients with confirmed paroxysms of arterial blood desaturation at night, and this also in cases whose resting values of blood gases are still within normal, for episodes of arterial blood desaturation are associated with paroxysms of pulmonary hypertension, as demonstrated by Boysen et al.[7] The hypertension is initially transient and is related to the severity and duration of desaturation.

The role of this factor in the development of chronic cor pulmonale is at present the subject of intensive study. There has been an effort recently to administer oxygen during nocturnal desaturation to prevent the onset and development of pulmonary hypertension.

An interesting study was conducted by DeOlbazal et al.[14] The Authors studied the incidence of nocturnal desaturation and cardiac dysrhythmias in a group of 17 middle-aged men with stable Ischaemic Heart Disease (IHD) documented by coronary angiography. Thirteen and 12 patients were found to have paroxysms of nocturnal desaturation and nocturnal dysrhythmia, respectively.

The study suggests the importance of research into this issue in patients with IHD. A trial with a design similar to ours was conducted by Tirlapur et al.[15] We were unable to find many such studies in the literature. The Authors studied the relationship between nocturnal hypoxaemia and the incidence of ECG alterations in a group of 12 patients with COLD. While seven patients showed prevalence of the BB type, the remaining ones were diagnosed as the PP type of COLD. In addition, the subjects were divided by their smoking status.

The results of this trial clearly demonstrated that patients with prevalent obstructive bronchitis have a higher incidence of cardiac dysrhythmias, higher heart rate during sleep, and a number of ECG alterations (prolonged QTc interval, ST-T depression, incomplete PRT blockade, etc.). Oxygen administration partly normalized these ECG changes.

The Authors assume that significant hypoxaemia (a SaO_2 below 80%) has a direct effect on the myocardium and produces an array of ECG changes in BB patients. However, it appears that even the beneficial effect of oxygen does not eliminate fully the risk of sudden death from dysrhythmias in patients who have not quit smoking. Previous studies did not demonstrate a statistically significant relationship between a decrease in paO_2 and the incidence of cardiac dysrhythmias.

However, this does not imply no such correlation really exists. To explain, single-dose, even though repeated, blood collection for blood gas analysis does not allow us to determine the elusive dynamics of nocturnal desaturation and increase in ectopic heart activity, which has been made possible only by the development of new non-invasive monitoring techniques in recent years, as just another beneficial aspect of these studies.

As has been said, the prognostic value of cardiac dysrhythmias in COLD is a most intriguing question.

In their study published in 1988, Shih et al.[16] report on a group of 69 patients treated with long-term oxygenotherapy. Using multifactorial analysis, they evaluated the prognosis of patients to find that not the dysrhythmias per se, but a medical history of ischaemic heart disease, increased heart rate and decreased physical fitness were the actual risk factors of death.

This, to a certain extent surprising, finding made recently underlines the necessity of further research regarding cardiac dysrhythmias in patients with advanced obstructive pulmonary disease. However, in the literature available to us, we did not find any reference to Holter findings in patients dying from cor pulmonale.

Conclusion

Our statistical data cannot be used to define the prognostic value of dysrhythmias in cor pulmonale. To be able to do so, further studies in larger groups of patients are required. Still, we do find our data most interesting and hope they might stimulate further research in this non-invasive technique in patients with chronic cor pulmonale.

1. A group of patients dying from cor pulmonale showed a higher incidence of atrial and ventricular dysrhythmias than a group of living subjects.

2. To assess the prognostic value of this finding, further studies in large groups of patients will be necessary.

3. There is no direct correlation between the incidence of cardiac dysrhythmias and arterial blood desaturation.

Despite this, both methods complement each other. There is an indirect correlation between resting paO_2 and the degree of exertional arterial blood desaturation. A significant correlation was demonstrated between the incidence of atrial dysrhythmias and arterial blood desaturation, but not the value of paO_2.

References

1. Brodsky M., et al.: Arrhythmia documented by 24-hour continuous ambulatory monitoring in 50 male students without apparent diseases. J. Am. Cardiol. 1977; 39:390-395
2. Clark P.I., Glasser S.P., Spote E.: Arrhythmias detected by ambulatory monitoring. Chest 1980; 77:722-725
3. Conradson T.B., et al.: Cardiac arrhythmias in patients with mild-to-moderate obstructive lung disease. Chest 1985; 88:537-542
4. Klieger R.E., Senior R.M.: Long-term electrocardiographic monitoring of ambulatory patients with chronic airway obstruction. Chest 1974; 65:483-487
5. Flick M.R., Block A.J.: Chronic oxygen therapy. Med. Clin. North Amer. 1977; 61:1397-1407
6. Holford F.D., Mithoefer J.C.: Cardiac arrhythmias in hospitalized patients with chronic obstructive pulmonary disease. Amer. Rev. Resp. Dis. 1973; 108:879-885
7. Boysen P.G.: Nocturnal pulmonary hypertension in patients with chronic obstructive pulmonary disease. Chest 1979; 76:536-541
8. DeMarco F.J., et al.: Oxygen desaturation during sleep as a determinant of the "blue and bloated" syndrome. Chest 1981; 79:821-825
9. Block A.J., Boysen P.B., Wayne J.W.: The origins of cor pulmonale. A hypothesis. Chest 1979; 75:109-110
10. Senior R.M., et al.: The heart in chronic obstructive disease. Arrhythmias. Chest 1979; 75:1-2
11. Ashutosh K., Dunsky M.: Noninvasive tests for responsiveness of pulmonary hypertension on oxygen. Chest 1987; 92:393-399
12. Josephson G.W.: Cardiac dysrhythmias during the treatment of acute asthma. Chest 1980; 429-435
13. Goren C., Dones P.: The role of Holter monitoring in detecting digitalis provoked arrhythmias. Chest, 1981; 555-558
14. De Olabazal J.R., et al.: Disordered breathing and hypoxia during sleep in coronary artery disease. Chest 1982; 82: 548-552
15. Tizlapur V.G. et al.: Nocturnal hypoxaemia and associated electrocardiographic changes in patients with chronic obstructive airways disease. New Eng. J. Med. 1982; 306:125-130
16. Shih Hue-Teh et al.: Frequency and significance of cardiac arrhythmias in chronic obstructive lung disease. Chest 1988; 94:44-48

15. Haemodynamics and Gas Exchange, Irrespective of Hypoxia, in Severe Obstructive Pulmonary Disease

A. Dees[1,3], P.N. Van Es[1], M. Heysteeg[2], P.W. de Leeuw[1]

1. Department of Internal Medicine, Zuiderziekenhuis, Rotterdam, Netherlands
2. Department of Pulmonary Medicine, Zuiderziekenhuis, Rotterdam, Netherlands
3. Department of Internal Medicine, Ikaziaziekenhuis, Rotterdam, Netherlands

Introduction

In recent years much attention has been paid to the role of pulmonary haemodynamics and right ventricular function in the course of hypoxic chronic obstructive pulmonary disease (COPD).[1] Pulmonary hypertension and cor pulmonale have been recognized as important prognostic factors.[2]

The survival and quality of life in hypoxic COPD are greatly improved by the introduction of long term oxygen therapy (LTOT) in the home care situation.[3,4] However, only a selected number of patients will benefit from LTOT and so the focus of interest has changed to the early diagnosis of pulmonary hypertension and right ventricular dysfunction.[5,6]

Apart from the evaluation of diagnostic tools, especially the noninvasive evaluation of right ventricular performance[7,8] there is a renewed interest into the pathophysiological mechanisms which underlie hypoxic cor pulmonale. Since oedema in hypoxic COPD is observed especially in patients with hypercapnia, the relationship of blood gas tensions to systemic haemodynamics requires further investigation.

Therefore, we decided to explore the relationship between pulmonary and systemic haemodynamics on the one hand, and gas exchange on the other in patients with advanced COPD, under conditions of normoxia.

Patients and Methods

Twenty-six consecutive patients with severe COPD, suspected of having pulmonary hypertension were studied. The selection of patients was based on clinical information, such as sustained hypoxia, hypercapnia, electrocardiographic signs of right ventricular hypertrophy and increased diameter of pulmonary arteries on chest X-ray. To exclude the influence of hypoxic drive on haemodynamics and cardiac performance, all investigations were carried out during normoxia. To this end patients with PaO_2 less than 60 mmHg at rest, received supplemental oxygen by nasal canulae, at least 24 hour prior to investigation. Baseline characteristics of the patients are shown in Table I.

Nearly all of them were heavy smokers and all were taking several drugs, including β-agonists, methylxanthines and corticosteroids. The drug regime remained unchanged throughout the study. In 11 patients medical history revealed one or more periods of oedema, but at the time of the study all were in stable condition, without signs of exacerbation or decompensated cor pulmonale. Patients were excluded from the study in case of systemic hypertension (Mean Arterial Pressure>110 mmHg) or when renal or hepatic disease was present. Patients with overt valvular or coronary heart disease were excluded as well.

Swan-Ganz thermodilution and radial artery catheters were inserted for haemodynamic measurements and sampling of blood. Measurements were made during steady state conditions with patients in supine position. Baseline haemodynamic data, were obtained after a stabilisation period of half an hour. The zero reference point for the pulmonary artery parameters was placed at mid chest, the cardiac output was measured with a cardiac output computer. Standard formulas were used for calculations of derived haemodynamic variables. Blood sampling of arterial and mixed venous blood was performed anaerobically.

Statistical methods applied were 2-way analysis of variance and t-tests. Data are expressed as mean ± standard deviation (SD). The study was reviewed and approved by the hospital ethical committee and patients gave informed consent.

Results

The baseline characteristics (Tab. I), demonstrate that patients were of older age with signs of severe obstructive lung disease. During supplemental oxygen therapy (mean FiO_2 24±3 percent) PaO_2 and MvO_2 (38±4 mmHg) were within the normal range, but mild hypercapnia was noted. Haemodynamic data (Tab. II) showed normal values for wedge pressure and mean arterial pressure. For the whole group of patients a number of haemodynamic variables were related to arterial carbon dioxide tension ($paCO_2$) as shown in figures 1-4. The RVSWI was related to MvO_2 (p=0.01) and $MvCO_2$ (p=0.0025) also.

The haematocrit showed weak relations to mPAP ($p<0.05$), pH ($p<0.05$) and PVR ($0.05<p<0.10$), but no clear relationships were found between paO_2 and the systemic or pulmonary haemodynamics. In 14 patients pulmonary hypertension, defined as mean pulmonary artery pressure (mPAP) >20 mmHg at rest, was found. These patients differed from the remainder in haematocrit (0.52±0.04vs

Table I. Patient characteristics

Age (years)	68.00±8.00	pH	7.40± 0.04
BSA (m²)	1.75±0.17	paO$_2$ (mmHg)	72.00±17.00
Hb (mmol.l^{-1})	10.10±0.80	paCO$_2$ (mmHg)	47.00± 8.00
Ht	0.50±0.04		
FEV$_1$ (1)	0.81±0.18		
FEV$_1$/FVC	0.34±0.08		

Table II. Haemodynamic data

	A (All patients)	B (Patients with mPAP ≤ 20 mmHg)	C (Patients with mPAP > 20 mmHg)	
Number	26	12	14	p*
mAP (mmHg)	92±13	88±16	95±11	NS
mRAP (mmHg)	3±2	3±1	4±3	NS
mPAP (mmHg)	23±9	16±3	28±8	<0.001
mPCWP (mmHg)	7±3	6±2	7±3	NS
HR (b.min^{-1})	88±14	83±14	91±13 0	NS
CI (l.min-1 .m^{-2})	3.12±0.62	3.19±0.63	3.06±0.62	NS
SVI (ml.beat-1 .m^{-2})	36 ±9	39±10	34±7	NS
SVR (dyne.sec.cm^{-5})	1363±294	1317±354	1403±239	NS
PVR (dyne.sec.cm^{-5})	243±121	156±32	318±120	<0.001
LVSWI				
(ml.mmHg.m^{-2})	3356±880	3458.00±1067	3270±714	NS
RVSWI (gm.m^{-2})	11.5±4.60	9.50±3.3	13.20±4.80	<0.05

* Denotes level of statistical significance between groups B and C

0.47±0.03; p<0.01), FEV$_1$/FVC (0.31±0.08 vs 0.37±0.07; p<0.05), pH (7.38±0.02 vs 7.42±0.02; p<0.05) and right ventricular stroke work index (13.2±4.8 vs 9.5±3.3; p<0.05). No statistical differences were found with respect to any of the other haemodynamic variables or to systemic oxygen transport.

Discussion

Before discussing the results of the present study a few remarks with respect to its design are in order. Usually studies in patients with hypoxic COPD are aimed

178

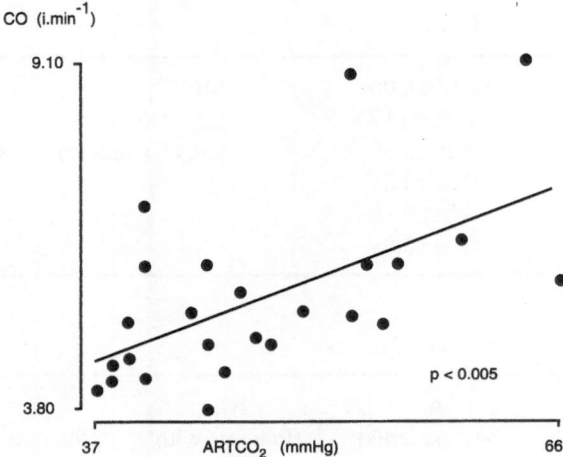

Fig. 1. Cardiac output in relation to arterial carbon dioxide tension.

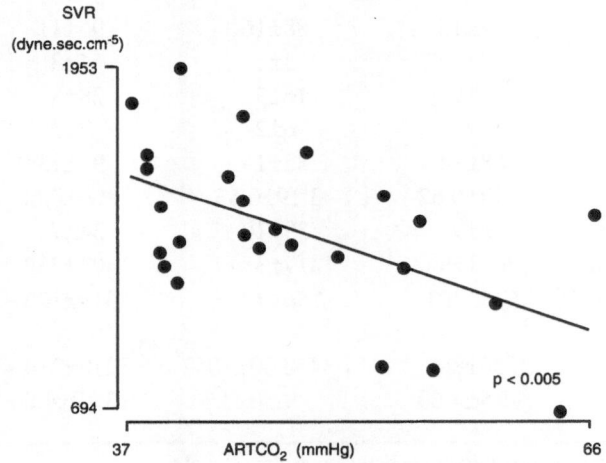

Fig. 2. Systemic vascular resistance in relation to arterial carbon dioxide tension.

at blunting vasoconstriction by means of oxygen or vasodilating agents.[9-12] Since vasoconstriction will occur both in chronic and acute hypoxia, the clinical condition of the patient and severity of hypoxaemia should be well defined.

Selinger has shown that withdrawal of oxygen in patients treated with LTOT, is followed by increases up to 30 percent in pulmonary artery pressure and pulmonary vascular resistance, which takes 2 to 3 hours to reach a new steady state and is a strong argument for the continuous use of LTOT.[13] For this reason, patients in the present study were treated with oxygen, for 24 hours prior to the investigation.

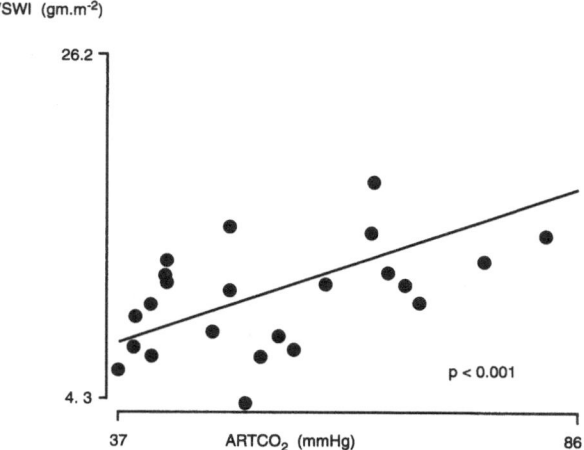

Fig. 3. Right ventricular stroke work index in relation to arterial carbon dioxide tension.

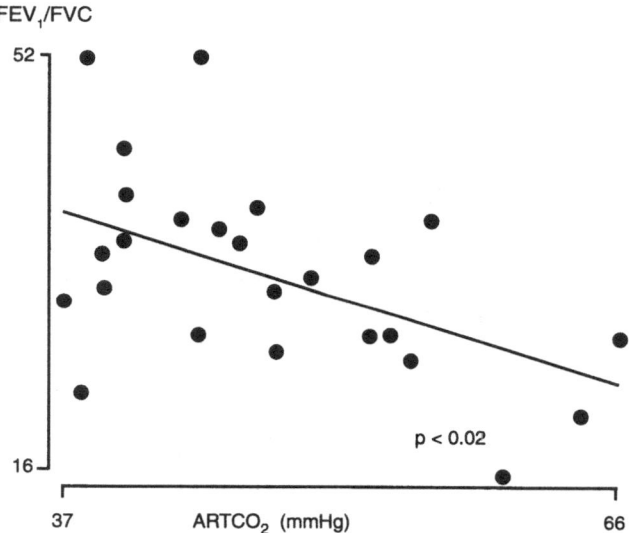

Fig. 4. One second forward expiratory volume/vital capacity in relation to arterial carbon dioxide tension.

Our data in patients with COPD show that, during normoxia, cardiac output is directly related to $paCO_2$ and systemic vascular resistance (SVR) inversely.

Several hypotheses may be put forward to explain these findings. Firstly, the induction of systemic vasodilation by hypercapnia may occur as a primary event, followed by a secondary rise in cardiac output. Indeed carbon dioxide is a potent vasodilator and an important factor in the autoregulation of vascular wall tension, especially in the cerebral vasculature.[14] After infusion of bicarbonate solution, as shown in a study with ventilated dogs[15], marked increases in cardiac output and decreases of SVR were observed, related to the change in $paCO_2$.

Selinger et al.[13] found that withdrawal of oxygen was followed by a decrease in oxygen transport and uptake in hypercapnic patients. However, normocapnic patients were able to increase oxygen consumption after withdrawal from LTOT. These data also suggest that in hypercapnic patients cardiac output is already enhanced.

A second possible explanation for the high cardiac output and low SVR in hypercapnic patients relates to a hyperdynamic circulation. In this view the rise in cardiac output could be caused by an increase in circulating blood volume. For instance renal retention of extracellular fluid, could lead to an increase in right ventricular preload and hence cardiac output. A high cardiac output state may also be secondary to increased venous return as a consequence of the negative intrathoracic pressure.

Both mechanisms have potentially important consequences. In this respect one could think of the decrease in right ventricular filling pressure during positive pressure ventilation[16] or the role of the kidney in the pathogenesis of oedema.[17-20]

In the present study no differences in cardiac output or SVR were noted between patients with and those without pulmonary hypertension, which is in agreement with previous studies.[5,9]

In conclusion, in this study marked vasodilation associated with hypercapnia during normoxia was observed. At this moment the question remains unanswered whether systemic vasodilation is beneficial or harmful to the hypercapnic patient. However, for practical reasons one should be aware of the haemodynamic setting in hypercapnic patients, in particular when prescribing vasodilating agents.

References

1. Weitzenblum E., Hirth C., Duculone A., Mirhom R., Rasaholinjanahary R., Ehrart M.: Prognostic value of pulmonary artery pressure in chronic obstructive pulmonary disease. Thorax 1981; 36:752-758
2. Finley M., Middeleton H.C., Peake M.D., Howard P.: Cardiac output, pulmonary hypertension, hypoxaemia and survival in patients with chronic obstructive airway disease. Eur. J. Resp. Dis. 1983; 38:498-500
3. Bardsley P.A., Howard P.: Cor pulmonale and home oxygen therapy. Practitioner 1986; 230:565-571
4. Weitzenblum E., Sautegeau A., Ehrhard M., Mammoser M., Pelletier A.: Longterm oxygen therapy can reverse the progression of pulmonary hypertension in patients with chronic obstructive pulmonary disease. Am. Rev. Resp. Dis. 1985; 131:493-498
5. Timms R.M., Khaja F.U., Williams G.W.: Haemodynamic response to oxygen therapy in chronic obstructive pulmonary disease. Ann. Int. Med. 1985; 102:29-36
6. Ashutosh K., Dunsky M.: Noninvasive tests for responsiveness of pulmonary hypertension to

oxygen. Prediction of survival in patients with chronic obstructive lung disease and cor pulmonale. Chest 1987; 92:393-399

7. Johnson R.A., Rubin L.J.: Noninvasive evaluation of right ventricular function. Clinics Chest Med. 1987; 8:65-80

8. Bishop J.M., Csukas M.: Combined use of non-invasive techniques to predict pulmonary artery pressure in chronic respiratory disease. Thorax 1989; 44:85-96

9. MacNee W., Wathen C.G., Flenley D.C., Muir A.D.: The effects of controlled oxygen therapy on ventricular function in patients with stable and decompensated cor pulmonale. Am. Rev. Resp. Dis. 1988; 1289-1295

10. Burke C.M., Horte M., Duncan J., Conally H.M., Morgan J.H.: Captopril and domiciliary oxygen in chronic airflow obstruction. Br. Med. J. 1985; 290:1251-1252

11. Treacher D.F., Douglas A., Jones A., Bateman N.T., Bradley R.D., Cameron I.R.: The acute hemodynamic effects of intravenous verapamil in patients with chronic obstructive airways disease. Quart. J. Med. 1987; 247:941-952

12. Kennedy T.P., Michael J.R., Huang C.K., et al.: Nifedipine inhibits hypoxic pulmonary vasoconstriction during rest and exercise in patients with chronic obstructive pulmonary disease: Am. Rev. Resp. Dis. 1984; 129:544-551

13. Selinger S.R., Kennedy T.P., Buescher P., et al.: Effects of removing oxygen from patients with chronic obstructive pulmonary disease. Am. Rev. Resp. Dis. 1987; 136:85-91

14. Detweiler D.K.: Circulation through brain, skin and skeletal muscle. In: Brosbeck J.R. (Ed) *Physiological basis of medical practice*. 9th ed. Baltimore, The Williams & Wilkins Company, 1973

15. Oddoy A., Danzmann E., Merker G., et al.: Acute effects of bicarbonate infusion on pulmonary and systemic haemodynamics in beagle dogs. Proceedings, International Symposium on Pulmonary Circulation V, Prague 1989

16. Assmann R., Falke K.J.: Pressure and volume assessment of right ventricular function during mechanical ventilation. Int. Care Med. 1988; 14 (suppl. 2):467-470

17. Stuart-Harris, Macinnon J., Hammond J.D.S., Smith W.D.: The renal circulation in chronic pulmonary disease and pulmonary heart failure. Q.J. Med. 1956; 25:389-405

18. Oliver R.M., Peacock A.J., Fleming J.S., Waller D.G.: Renal and pulmonary effects of angiotensin converting enzyme inhibition in chronic hypoxic lung disease. Thorax 1989; 44:513-515

19. Farber M.O., Manfredi F.: Mechanisms of hyponatremia and edema in chronic obstructive pulmonary disease: clinical significance. Pract Cardiol. 1984; 10:105-131

20. Editorial. What causes oedema. Lancet, 1988; 1:1028-1030

16. Pulmonary Haemodynamics in "Pure" Emphysema

M.O. Mammosser, M. Apprill, R. Mirhom, M. Ehrhart, E. Weitzenblum

Pulmonary Function Laboratory, Pavillon Laennec, University Hospital, Strasbourg, France

Introduction

Pulmonary hypertension (PH) leading to clinical "cor pulmonale" is often observed in patients with advanced chronic obstructive pulmonary disease (COPD).[1,2] In fact, PH occurs mostly in COPD patients of the "bronchitic" type, the so-called "blue and bloated" patients.[3,4] It is less frequently observed in "pink puffer" patients of the "emphysematous" type.[5,7] However, "pink puffer" is not synonymous with emphysematous, and a recent study[8] has clearly shown that the correlation between the morphological grade of emphysema and the degree of hypoxaemia, hypercapnia and pulmonary hypertension was rather poor.

Most haemodynamic studies have dealt with COPD patients of the "bronchitic" type.[5,9-12] To our knowledge very few studies have been devoted to patients with "pure" or predominant emphysema.[6,13,14]

It is generally accepted that chronic alveolar hypoxia is the determining factor of PH in COPD patients.[15] Hypoxaemia is classically mild or absent in emphysematous patients.[6,7]

Is PH similarly rare or absent in these patients? If this is not the case, what are the causes of pulmonary haemodynamic abnormalities in emphysematous patients? We therefore found it of interest to investigate pulmonary haemodynamics, at rest and during exercise, in a large series (n=151) of "predominantly" or "purely" emphysematous patients. The aim of the present study was to assess the frequency and the possible mechanisms of PH in these patients. Particular attention was paid to patients with diffuse emphysema plus large compressive bullae since specific haemodynamic abnormalities have been described in this subgroup of patients[16] which need further confirmation.

Methods

One hundred and fifty-one patients were included in this retrospective study. There were 148 males and 3 females, age averaging 58.4±9.7 years (19-81 years). Emphysema was assessed on clinical, radiological and functional grounds.

Dyspnoea was the major complaint of the patients; cough and sputum were absent or of little importance. The classical radiological signs of emphysema[17] were required: pulmonary distension, vascular scarcity, flat and lowered diaphragms.

The presence of emphysematous bullae was not an obligatory criterion but was carefully assessed. CT scans were available in very few patients since most investigations were performed at a time before this investigation was readily available.

Functional criteria of emphysema were: increased residual volume (RV), total lung capacity (TLC) and residual volume to TLC ratio; and an obstructive spirographic pattern (decreased $FEV_1/VC: \leq 60\%$). Despite the fact that anatomical confirmation of emphysema, by necropsy or thoracic surgery, was available in a rather limited number of cases, there is no doubt that emphysema (of some degree) was present in all cases and was the predominant feature of COPD.

Twenty patients had diffuse pulmonary emphysema plus large "compressive" bullae. They were included in the whole group for statistical analysis but they were also analysed separately in order to examine the behaviour of such patients from rest to exercise.

All patients were investigated in a stable state of their disease. Those having cardiovascular disturbances other than those related to pulmonary emphysema (systemic hypertension, left heart diseases) were excluded from the study. We also excluded patients with pulmonary carcinoma and sequelae of pulmonary tuberculosis.

Static pulmonary volumes (FRC, TLC) were measured by the helium dilution method in a closed circuit. Vital capacity (VC) and FEV_1 were measured with a ten-litre closed circuit spirograph. The transfer factor for carbon monoxide (TLCO) was measured using the single-breath method in 66 patients (alveolo-diffusion test Jaeger). In 27 additional patients the transfer factor for oxygen (TLO_2) was measured with a method described elsewhere.[18]

Right heart catheterization was performed as described earlier:[19] patients were investigated in the supine position in the morning without premedication; the zero reference level for vascular pressure was taken as 7.5 cm below the sternal angle.

Pressures were obtained with a Grandjean F_4 Flexopulmocath[20] introduced in a peripheral vein (in most cases a basilic vein, in some instances by femoral catheterization). Exercise was performed in the supine position on an ergometric bicycle; the load was of 40 watts or less. The exercise test lasted 8-10 minutes in order to obtain a steady state. Pulmonary wedge pressure (PWP) could be obtained in 114 cases at rest and in 75 cases during exercise. Cardiac output (CO) was measured using the Fick's method applied to oxygen, the O_2 uptake being measured with a Fleisch closed circuit metabograph.

Pulmonary vascular resistance (PVR) could be calculated in 89 cases at rest and 49 cases during exercise, by the formula:

$$PVR = \frac{PAP\text{-}PWP}{CO}$$

where PAP is the pulmonary artery mean pressure.

We also measured the amplitude of the respiratory swings of the diastolic PAP (ΔPd) during quiet breathing. During catheterization blood samples were obtained from a brachial artery through a Cournand needle and from the pulmonary artery in order to measure PaO_2, $PaCO_2$, SaO_2, pH and PvO_2. The alveolar PO_2 (PaO_2) was obtained by the ideal alveolar air equation[21] and this allowed the calculation of the alveolar-arterial PO_2 difference ($AaDO_2$).

Statistical analysis

Comparisons between the means were made by Student's t-test for large groups ($n\geq30$) and by the Wilcoxon test for smaller groups ($n<30$). Multiple regression was performed using the step by step regression analysis. The level of statistical significance was $p<0.05$.

Results

The functional data are presented in Table I. It can be observed that bronchial obstruction was generally moderate to severe with a mean FEV_1 of 1.2 ± 0.6 litre and a mean FEV_1/VC ratio of $38.2\pm12.4\%$. As expected, RV and RV/TLC ratio were markedly increased. The transfer factor was moderately decreased as a mean. Only few patients had mild functional disturbances.

In Tables II and III are summarized the average arterial blood gases (ABG) and the average haemodynamic data. The ABG measurements showed mild hypoxaemia at rest and during exercise (no significant difference for PaO_2 between rest and exercise) without hypercapnia. $PaCO_2$ increased significantly ($p < 0.0005$) from rest (37.2 ± 5.0 mmHg) to exercise (40.1 ± 6.4 mmHg). Pulmonary hypertension (PH) (defined by a $PAP\geq20$ mmHg) was present in only 31/151 patients (20.5% of the cases), and the average value for the group was 17.1 ± 5 mmHg. During steady state exercise an abnormally high $\overline{PAP}$ (≥30 mmHg) was observed in 99/151 patients (65.6% of the cases), the average $\overline{PAP}$ being of 34.3 ± 9.9 mmHg. PWP rose from 6.3 ± 2.0 mmHg at rest to 14.3 ± 4.8 mmHg during exercise. None of the patients had an abnormally high PWP (>12 mmHg) at rest and in only 6/75 cases was PWP higher than 20 mmHg during exercise. Above these threshold values, PWP is

Table I. Functional data of the 151 emphysematous patients

Variables	Number	Mean	SD	Max.	Min.
VC	151	3.09	0.82	6.15	1.20
VC (% of predicted)	151	81.2	18.8	146	36.9
RV	151	3.66	1.03	6.37	1.43
RV/TLC (%)	151	53.4	10.5	81.6	25.6
FEV$_1$ (l)	151	1.20	0.59	4.10	0.45
FEV$_1$/VC (%)	151	38.2	12.4	60	17.3
TLCO (ml/mmHg/min)	66	18.1	7.3	38.4	5.05
TLCO (% of predicted)	66	70.3	26.5	146.5	18.5
TLO$_2$ (ml/mmHg/min)	27	13.3	11.4	61.6	5.2

VC = vital capacity;   TLO$_2$ = O$_2$ transfer factor;
RV = residual volume;   Max. = maximal value;
TLC = total lung capacity;   Min. = minimal value;
TLCO = CO transfer factor;   SD= standard deviation.

Table II. Arterial blood gases data of the 151 patients

	Number	Mean	SD	Max.	Min.
PaO$_2$r (mmHg)	151	70.9	11.2	112	34
PaO$_2$e (mmHg)	150	70.0	13.2	109	42
PaCO$_2$r (mmHg)	151	37.2	5.0	53	27.5
PaCO$_2$e (mmHg)	150	40.1	6.4	66.5	29
AaDO$_2$r (mmHg)	102	37.7	10.6	58.5	6.4
AaDO$_2$e (mmHg)	97	31.1	13.2	61.4	0

r = rest; e = exercise; SD= standard deviation

generally considered as being abnormally high.[22] Cardiac index was generally normal at rest (3.3±0.9 l/min/m^2) and increased as expected in normal subjects for the level of exercise performed to 6.6±2.1 l/min/m^2. In 49 patients PVR could be calculated both at rest and during exercise. PVR was moderately elevated at rest (1.8±0.7 mmHg/l/min) and did not change during exercise (1.7±0.9 mmHg/l/min).

Table III. Haemodynamic data of the 151 patients

Variables	Number	Mean	SD	Max.	Min.
$\overline{PAPr}$ (mmHg)	151	17.1	5.0	40	9.5
PAPe (mmHg)	151	34.3	9.9	70	15
PWPr (mmHg)	114	6.3	2.0	11	1.5
PWPe (mmHg)	75	14.3	4.8	30	5
PVRr (units)	89	2.0	1.0	7.5	0.4
PVRe (units	49	1.7	0.9	5.2	0.5
CIr (l/min/m^2)	117	3.3	0.9	6.2	1.6
CIe (l/min/m^2)	98	6.6	2.1	16.3	3.2

PAPr = pulmonary artery mean pressure at rest;
PAPe = pulmonary artery mean pressure during exercise;
PWPr = pulmonary wedge pressure at rest;
PWPe = pulmonary wedge pressure during exercise;
PVRr = pulmonary vascular resistance at rest;
PVRe = pulmonary vascular resistance during exercise;
CIr = cardiac index at rest;
CIe = cardiac index during exercise
SD: standard deviation

21 patients exhibited marked hypoxaemia (PaO_2 ≤60 mmHg). Their average functional, ABG and haemodynamic data as well as those of the others (n=130) are presented in Tables IV and V. Hypoxaemic patients differed from the others with regard to their functional data (particularly FEV_1 and FEV_1/VC) and $\overline{PAP}$ at rest. By definition these patients were more hypoxaemic at rest; PaO_2 and $PaCO_2$ both increased significantly (p<0.05) during exercise. Resting PWP was 6.5±2.9 mmHg (n=15) and exercising PWP was 13.9±3.7 mmHg (n=8). CI (n=17) increased

Table IV. Functional data in patients with and without hypoxaemia

Variables	VC (% predicted)	RV/TLC (%)	FEV_1 (l)	FEV_1/VC (%)
Hypoxaemic (n=21)	73.2±20.3	58.4±10.9	0.94±0.35	34.0±7.0
Remainders (n=130)	82.6±18.2	52.6±10.3	1.24±0.61	38.4±13.1
p value	<0.05	<0.01	<0.001	<0.001

For abbreviations see Tables I-III. Values are expressed as mean±SD

Table V. Arterial blood gases and haemodynamic data in patients with and without hypoxaemia

Variables	PaO$_2$r (mmHg)	PaO$_2$e (mmHg)	PaCO$_2$r (mmHg)	PaCO$_2$e (mmHg)	PAPr (mmHg)	PAPe (mmHg)
Hypoxaemic (n = 21)	54.4±6.1	61.2±13.5	39.5±5.9	43.2±9.5	19±4.7	37.3±9.1
Others (n = 130)	73.6±9.3	71.6±12.6	36.8±4.8	39.6±5.6	16.8±4.9	33.9±10.0
p value	p<0.001	p<0.001	p<0.05	NS	p<0.02	NS

For abbreviations see Tables I-III. Values are expressed as mean ± 1SD

normally from rest (3.6±1.1 l/min/m^2) to exercise (6.4±2.3 l/min/m^2).

Thirty-one patients had resting PH. Their average functional, ABG and haemodynamic data as well as those of the others (n=120) are presented in Tables VI and VII. Hypertensive patients differed from the others with regard to RV/TLC, FEV$_1$ and FEV$_1$/VC. These indexes indicated more obstruction and pulmonary distension in patients with PH. But the latter did not differ from the non-hypertensive patients with regard to PaO$_2$ at rest. During exercise PaO$_2$ decreased significantly (p<0.001) and was markedly lower than in non-hypertensive patients. By definition PAP at rest was increased and showed a further important increase during exercise. In 17 hypertensive patients CI could be calculated at rest and during exercise. It increased from 3.2±1.0 at rest to 5.5±1.3 l/min/m^2 during exercise. PWP at rest was 7.8±2.1 mmHg (n=24) and 16.1 ± 3.2 mmHg (n=15) during exercise.

In the twenty patients with large "compressive" bullae, PAP increased from 17.5 ± 4.1 mmHg at rest to 33.6 ± 9.6 mmHg during exercise. CI could be measured in 11 patients at rest and during exercise, it increased from 3.1±0.7 to 6.5±1.9 l/min/

Table VI. Functional data in patients with and without pulmonary hypertension

Variables	VC (% predicted)	RV/TLC (%)	FEV$_1$ (l)	FEV$_1$/VC (%)
Pulmonary hypertension (n=31)	78.2±17.1	56.1±8.5	0.92±0.29	32.2±6.9
Others (n = 120)	82.1±19.2	53.6±14.2	1.27±0.63	39.8±13.0
p value	NS	<0.01	<0.001	<0.001

For abbreviations see Tables I-III. Values are expressed as mean ± 1SD

Table VII. Arterial blood gases and haemodynamic data in patients with and without pulmonary hypertension

Variables	PaO_2r (mmHg)	PaO_2e (mmHg)	$PaCO_2r$ (mmHg)	$PaCO_2e$ (mmHg)	PAPr (mmHg)	PAPe (mmHg)
Pulmonary hypertension (n=31)	68.4±13.5	60.9±13.7	40.0±5.7	44.2±7.8	24.6±4.8	45.7±9.7
Others (n=120)	71.6±9.8	72.4±12.1	36.6±4.9	39.1±5.5	15.2±2.6	31.4±7.6
p value	NS	<0.001	<0.001	<0.001	<0.001	<0.001

For abbreviations see Tables I-III. Values are expressed as mean ± 1SD

m^2. The correlations between $\overline{PAP}$ at rest and during exercise and functional and ABG data are presented in Table VIII. Resting $\overline{PAP}$ showed a rather weak correlation with PaO_2r but the correlations were stronger with ΔPd, TLCO and PaO_2e. Exercise $\overline{PAP}$ was correlated with TLCO, ΔPd, FEV_1 and PaO_2e. In the subgroup of patients with resting PH, $\overline{PAP}$ at rest was not correlated with PaO_2r but with PaO_2e (r = - 0.38; p < 0.05). We observed no correlation between $\overline{PAP}$ and other functional or ABG variables in this subgroup. In the patients with marked hypoxaemia, resting $\overline{PAP}$ was only correlated with PaO_2e (r = - 0.48; p<0.05).

Finally we analysed the predictive value of functional data and ABG variables by a step by step regression analysis (Table IX). The standard error was nearly the

Table VIII. Correlations

	$\overline{PAP}$ rest			$\overline{PAP}$ exercise		
	r	p	n	r	p	n
PaO_2r	-0.22	0.01	151	-0.12	NS	151
PaO_2e	-0.45	0.001	150	-0.35	0.001	150
$PaCO_2r$	0.31	0.001	151	0.61	0.05	151
$PaCO_2e$	0.30	0.001	150	0.23	0.01	150
ΔPd	0.36	0.001	146	0.36	0.001	146
FEV_1	-0.30	0.00	150	0.35	0.001	150
$AaDO_2$	0.28	0.001	97	0.39	0.001	97
TLCO	-0.37	0.01	66	-0.44	0.001	66

For abbreviations see Tables I-III. r = coefficient of correlation

Table IX. Step by step regression analysis

Including TLCO in the analysis: n = 60

Predictive equations	r	p	standard error (mmHg)
$\overline{PAPr} = 25.08 - 0.13 \ PaO_2e + 0.35 \ PaCO_2r$ $0.002 \ RV - 0.065 \ TLCO \ (\%)$	- 0.68	<0.001	4.4
$\overline{PAPe} = 72.96 - 0.004 \ RV - 0.396 \ FEV_1/VC$ $0.125 \ TLCO \ (\%)$	- 0.59	<0.001	9

Excluding TLCO from the analysis: n = 134

Predictive equations	r	p	standard error (mmHg)
$\overline{PAPr} = 18.9 - 0.13 \ PaO_2e + 0.23 \ PaCO_2r$ $- 0.001 \ RV + 0.24 \ \Delta Pd$	0.57	<0.001	4.1
$\overline{PAPe} = 42.7 - 0.20 \ PaO_2e + 0.49 \ \Delta Pd$	0.43	<0.001	9.2

For abbreviations see Tables I-III.

same for $\overline{PAPr}$ or $\overline{PAPe}$ when including TLCO in the analysis or when excluding this variable in order to obtain a larger series.

Discussion

Emphysema can only be assessed on morphological criteria and this holds particularly true for mild or "incipient" emphysema. In our patients with advanced COPD the diagnosis of emphysema was highly probable in the presence of typical radiological and functional abnormalities. Furthermore our patients exhibited the clinical and ABG features of the "emphysematous" or "pink puffer" type of COPD. It ensues that our series was fairly representative of "pure" or at least "predominant" emphysematous COPD, despite the fact that morphological and CT data could not be obtained in most of the cases.

Our results clearly indicate that PH is not the rule in patients with "pure" or "predominant" emphysema since it was observed in only 20% of the cases. This could be explained easily if many patients had mild emphysema but in fact this was not the case. It must be emphasized that emphysema was advanced in most of the cases, as illustrated by the average values of pulmonary function data (Tab. I). This means that emphysema does not necessarily lead to "cor pulmonale" even when functional impairment, including bronchial obstruction, is severe. In this regard there is a marked difference between COPD patients of the "emphysematous" and "bronchitic" type, the latter exhibiting PH earlier and more frequently.[5,7] Indeed this difference can be attributed to the more severe hypoxaemia observed in the patients of the "bronchitic" type.[7] Chronic alveolar hypoxia is known to be the major cause of PH in COPD patients[1,23] and it is clear that hypoxaemia was mild or absent in our large series of emphysematous patients, the average PaO_2 being 70.9 ± 11.2 mmHg, in spite of a rather severe degree of bronchial obstruction (average $FEV_1 =1.20\pm0.59$ l, average $FEV_1/VC=38.2\pm12.4$ %). Hypoxaemia is generally more pronounced in "bronchitic" patients exhibiting the same degree of obstructive pattern.[6,7]

Thus, the first explanation of our haemodynamic findings seems to be the presence of marked hypoxaemia in only a minority of patients.

But when we consider the two small subgroups with either PH (n=31) or significant hypoxaemia defined by a $PaO_2 \leq60$ mmHg (n=21), it appears that chronic hypoxaemia is probably not a determining factor of PH. Although $\overline{PAP}$ was significantly higher in the hypoxaemic group than in the remaining patients, PaO_2 was not significantly lower in the PH group than in the others: and we have observed only a weak correlation between PaO_2 and $\overline{PAP}$ in the group of 151 patients taken as a whole and no correlation at all between PaO_2r and $\overline{PAP}r$ in the two subgroups considered above. Our results could support the recent hypothesis of Reid[24] who stated that in "severe panacinar emphysema the precapillary unit is destroyed so that the pattern of response observed in hypoxaemia does not in fact occur". Thus, our data could fit in with two hypotheses which do not necessarily exclude each other.

First hypothesis: PH is rarely observed in emphysematous patients because hypoxaemia is mild or absent. The lack of correlation between PaO_2 and $\overline{PAP}$ could be explained by the restricted number of patients with either an abnormally high PAP (≥ 20 mmHg) or a low PaO_2 (≤ 60 mmHg).

Second hypothesis: in panacinar emphysema, the frequency of which cannot be appreciated in our patients, alveolar hypoxaemia, even if present, could not induce PH since the precapillary unit, where the haemodynamic response to alveolar hypoxia takes place[15], is destroyed. This could account for the lack of a good correlation between PaO_2r and $\overline{PAP}r$.

That PH was rarely present at rest but occurred in two thirds of the patients during exercise, could be due to the anatomical amputation of the pulmonary vascular bed. We know from pulmonary thrombo-embolic disease that such an amputation must be higher than 50-60% to induce resting PH,[25] but PH is more likely to occur during exercise due to the increased cardiac output. In our patients cardiac index increased by nearly 100% of its resting value during steady state exercise. As pulmonary vascular resistance (PVR) was hardly changed, this resulted in an increase of $\overline{PAP}$ by about 100% of the baseline value at rest. In healthy subjects PVR generally decreases during exercise due to the distention of the pulmonary vascular bed and the recruitment of additional vessels, but this cannot occur in emphysema which is characterized by a more or less pronounced destruction of the pulmonary microvasculature. We were not able to assess the extent of this amputation in our patients since we did not perform pulmonary angiograms.

In emphysematous patients the decreased single breath CO transfer factor is related, at least partly, to the reduction of the pulmonary vascular bed. Good correlations have been observed between TLCO and the anatomic extent of emphysema[26] and very recently Biernacki et al.[8] have found a highly significant correlation between TLCO/VA and density histogram assessed by CT scan. Thus, TLCO is an indicator of the degree of amputation of the pulmonary vascular bed and we have observed a significant correlation ($p < 0.001$) between TLCO and both resting and exercising PAP. However, the correlation coefficients were rather weak ($r = 0.37$ and $r = -0.44$ respectively), which is probably accounted for by the fact that TLCO does not only reflect the volume of the pulmonary microvascular bed in these patients.

In our opinion the presence of rather good correlations between exercising PaO_2 and resting and exercising PAP, whereas the correlations with resting PaO_2 were not significant at all, is an additional argument for the determining role of a reduced pulmonary vascular bed. It is accepted that exercising hypoxaemia is partly explained, in emphysematous patients, by a shortened transit time of the red cells in the pulmonary capillaries.[26] This shortening is due to the passage of a normal cardiac output through a reduced capillary bed. It ensues that exercising PaO_2 reflects the degree of amputation of the pulmonary capillary bed and this probably explains why PaO_2 during exercise is correlated with the pulmonary artery pressure.

Large respiratory pressure swings are usually observed in these patients. Marked intrathoracic pressure variations could favour the increase of PVR and $\overline{PAP}$[9,10,27] by inducing a functional compression of the pulmonary vascular bed.[9] In the present study significant correlations between the amplitude of the respiratory pressure swings (ΔPd) and PAP have been observed and it is of interest to note that the only significant differences between patients with and without PH related to FEV_1, FEV_1/VC and RV/TLC. Large intrathoracic pressure variations are a direct consequence of bronchial obstruction. Lockhart and al.[10] have suggested that the rise in pulmonary artery wedge pressure, during exercise, in COPD patients is due to the effects of these intrathoracic pressure swings and of the resulting increased load of the left ventricle. They have observed a close relationship between wedge pressure and $\overline{PAP}$ during exercise. Our findings were rather different and an abnormally high wedge pressure during exercise (> 20 mmHg) was observed in very few patients. Our data do not support the hypothesis that a left ventricular dysfunction plays a role in exercising PH.

It thus appears that the reduction of the pulmonary vascular bed is the major cause of pulmonary haemodynamic abnormalities, and that anatomical factors could contribute to the increased PVR and PAP, especially during exercise.

In this large series of emphysematous patients cardiac output was generally normal at rest and increased, as expected in normal subjects, during exercise. In some earlier studies cardiac index has been found to be low in emphysematous patients[5,28] but this was not confirmed by other studies.[13] In fact the "low output" pattern described by Burrows et al.[5] refers more to the clinical and ABG picture of "pink puffer" than to emphysema assessed on radiological and morphological grounds.

It has been observed, at least by one group[16], that cardiac output could not increase adequately with exercise in emphysematous patients exhibiting large "compressive" bullae. This particular behaviour has been attributed to the limitation of venous return due to the compression of the large intrathoracic vessels during expiration. In our subgroup of patients with large bullae cardiac index increased normally from rest to exercise in all individual cases. We have not observed any "emphysematous collapse" leading to a marked dysfunction of the cardiac pump during exercise, perhaps because the bullae were not large enough to induce cardiac and mediastinal compression.

Finally, $\overline{PAP}$ could not be satisfactorily predicted by any functional variable or even by a combination of variables, which can be explained by the multifactorial nature of PH in emphysema, and also by the fact that the degree of destruction of the pulmonary vascular bed was not accurately taken into account by any of these variables.

References

1. Fishman A.P.: Chronic cor pulmonale. State of the art. Am. Rev. Resp. Dis. 1976; 114:775-794
2. Ferrer M.I.: Cor pulmonale (pulmonary heart disease): present-day status. Am. Heart J. 1975; 89: 657-664
3. Dornhorst A.C.: Respiratory insufficiency. Lancet 1955; 1: 1105-1187
4. Mitchell R.S., Vincent T.N., Ryan S., Filley F.G.: Chronic obstructive bronchopulmonary disease. IV. The clinical and physiological differentiation of chronic bronchitis and emphysema. Am. J. Med. Sci. 1964; 247:513
5. Burrows B., Kettel L.J., Niden A.H., Rabinowitz M., Diener C.F.: Patterns of cardiovascular dysfunction in chronic obstructive lung disease. New Engl. J. Med. 1972; 286:912-918
6. Burrows B., Fletcher C.M., Heard B.E., Jones N.L., Wootliff J.S.: The emphysematous and bronchial type of chronic airway obstruction. Lancet 1966; 1:830-835
7. Weitzenblum E., Roeslin N., Hirth C., Oudet P.: Etude comparative des données cliniques et de la fonction respiratoire entre la bronchite chronique et l'emphysème "primitif". Respiration 1970; 27:493-510

8. Biernacki W., Gould G.A., Whyte K.F., Flenley D.C.: Pulmonary hemodynamics, gas exchange and the severity of emphysema as assessed by quantitative CT scan in chronic bronchitis and emphysema. Am. Rev. Respir. Dis. 1989; 139:1509-1515

9. Lockhart A., Tzareva M., Nader F., Leblanc P., Schrijen F., Sadoul P.: Elevated pulmonary artery wedge pressure at rest and during exercise in chronic bronchitis: fact or fancy. Clin. Sci. 1969; 37:503-517

10. Lockhart A., Nader F., Tzareva M., Schrijen F.: Comparative effects of exercise and isocapnic voluntary hyperventilation on pulmonary haemodynamics in chronic bronchitis and emphysema. Europ. J. Clin. Invest. 1970; 1:69-76

11. Emirgil C., Sobol B.J., Herbert W.H., Trout K.W.: Routine pulmonary function studies as a key to the status of the lesser circulation in chronic obstructive pulmonary disease. Am. J. Med. 1971; 50:191-199

12. Weitzenblum E., El Gharbi T., Vandevenne A., Bleger A., Hirth C., Oudet P.: Le comportement hémodynamique au cours de l'exercice musculaire dans la bronchite chronique non "décompensée". Bull. Physiopath. Resp. 1972; 8:49-71

13. Williams J.F.Jr., Behnke R.H.: The effect of pulmonary emphysema upon cardio-pulmonary hemodynamics at rest and during exercise. Ann. Int. Med. 1964; 60:824-834

14. Meunier-Carus J., Bogui P., Lampert E., Sautejau A.: L'hypertension artérielle pulmonaire des emphysémateux. Rev. Pneumol. Clin. 1987; 43:312-321

15. Fishman A.P.: Hypoxia on the pulmonary circulation. How and where it acts. Circulation Res. 1976; 38:221-231

16. Even P., Sors H., Safran D., Reynaud P., Venet A., Debesse B.: Hémodynamique des bulles d'emhysème, un nouveau syndrome: la tamponade cardiaque emphysémateuse. Rev. Fr. Mal. Resp. 1980; 8:117-120

17. Simon G.: *Principles of chest X-Ray diagnosis*. 4th ed. London, Butterworth, 1978

18. Weitzenblum E., Roeslin N., Hirth C., Vandevenne A., Oudet P.: La capacité de diffusion de l'oxygène dans l'insuffisance respiratoire chronique. J. Franç. Méd. Chir. Thor. 1970; 24:821-835

19. Weitzenblum E., Loiseau A., Hirth C., Mirhom R., Rasaholinjanahary J.: Course of pulmonary hemodynamics in patients with chronic obstructive pulmonary disease. Chest 1979; 75:656-662

20. Grandjean T.: Une microtechnique du cathétérisme cardiaque droit praticable au lit du malade sans contrôle radioscopique. Cardiologia (Basel) 1968; 51:184-192

21. Fenn N.O., Rahn H., Otis A.B.: A theoretical study of the composition of alveolar air altitude. Am. J. Physiol. 1946; 146:637-653

22. Tartulier M., Bourret M., Deyrieux F.: Les pressions artérielles pulmonaires chez l'homme normal. Effet de l'âge et de l'exercice musculaire. Bull. Physiopath. Resp. 1972; 8:1295-1321

23. Mitchell R.S., Ryan S., Petty T.L., Filley F.G.: The significance of morphological chronic hyperplastic bronchitis. Am. Rev. Resp. Dis. 1966; 93:720

24. Reid L.M.: Structure and function in pulmonary hypertension. New perceptions. Chest 1986; 89:279-288

25. Widimsky J.: The mechanism of pulmonary hypertension in pulmonary embolism. Bull. Physiopath. Resp. 1970; 6:147-184

26. Bates D.V., Macklem P.T., Christie R.V.: *Respiratory function in disease*. 2nd ed., Philadelphia, W.B. Saunders Company, 1971; 584 p.

27. Harris P., Segel N., Green I.: The influence of the airways resistance and alveolar pressure on the pulmonary vascular resistance in chronic bronchitis. Cardiovasc. Res. 1968; 2:84-92

28. Blount S.G.Jr.: Cardiac output in pulmonary emphysema. In: W.R. Adams, I. Vieth (Eds.) *Pulmonary circulation*. New York, Grune and Stratton Inc. 1959; pp. 160-170

17. Determinants of Echo-Doppler Indices of Left Ventricular Filling in Patients with Chronic Lung Diseases

A. Torbicki[1], I. Hawrylkiewicz[2], Z. Miskiewicz[1], T. Pasierski[1], K. Skwarski[2], R. Tramarin[3], J. Zielinski[2]

1. *Department of Hypertension and Angiology, Academy of Medicine , Warsaw, Poland*
2. *Department of Respiratory Medicine, Institute of Tuberculosis and Lung Diseases, University Hospital, Warsaw, Poland*
3. *Division of Cardiology, Clinica del Lavoro Foundation, Institute of Care and Research, Medical Center of Rehabilitation, Montescano, Pavia, Italy*

Introduction

Consequences of chronic lung diseases on left ventricular (LV) diastolic function have not been extensively studied.[1] Recent communications suggested, that LV filling in patients with COPD may be abnormal.[2,3] Louie et al. using Doppler echocardiography found evidence of left ventricular (LV) diastolic dysfunction in patients with primary pulmonary hypertension.[4]

The suggested mechanism was that of ventricular interdependence, causing restriction of left ventricular filling by the leftward displacement of the interventricular septum early in diastole. Using pulsed wave Doppler and M-mode echocardiography we found abnormal left ventricular filling also in many patients with chronic lung diseases despite only moderate elevation of pulmonary artery pressure when compared with the population studied by Louie.[4]

To confirm our observations and to approach the mechanisms responsible for this phenomenon we evaluated a number of variables which might have influenced the pattern of left ventricular filling in patients with chronic lung diseases.

Materials and Methods

The patients were recruited among those who were referred for right heart catheterization in order to evaluate the haemodynamic complications of their chronic lung disease. All the patients were in clinically stable conditions, without exacerbation of their pulmonary disease, which was confirmed by stable arterial blood gases.

The patients were free from arrhythmias and clinical signs of heart failure. Patients with systemic hypertension were excluded from the study. Special care was taken to analyse the history and ECG of the patients for symptoms referable to ischaemic heart disease. However, neither myocardial scintigraphy nor coronary angiographic examination were available. Measurements of left ventricular free wall thickness were attempted in all the patients to exclude its hypertrophy. Patients with pulmonary sarcoidosis, diabetes and other diseases known to affect left ventricular diastolic function were discarded. No age limit was set.

Within 48 hours after haemodynamic study the patients were submitted to pulsed wave Doppler and M-mode echocardiographic examination. Recordings were performed at a sweep speed of 100mm/sec during quiet respiration with simultaneously displayed chest plethysmographic tracing. All echo and Doppler measurements were taken at end-expiration and averaged over at least 4 respiratory cycles. Left and right ventricular diastolic dimensions (LVEDD, RVEDD) were measured. Left ventricular filling pattern was assessed on the basis of the ratio of peak blood flow velocity early in diastole to peak blood flow velocity during atrial contraction (E/A vel) at the level of the mitral valve (Fig. 1).

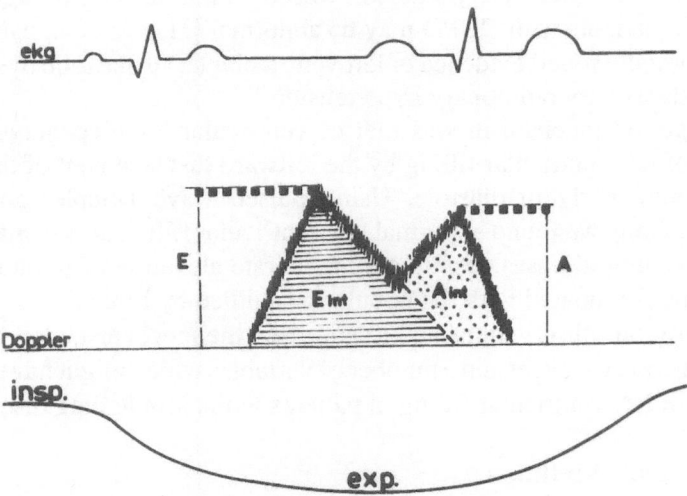

Fig. 1. Pulsed wave Doppler tracing of the mitral valve flow velocity: E - maximal early diastolic velocity, A - maximal velocity at atrial systole. The measurements of velocities and integrals under the velocity curves (Eint, Aint) were performed using the middle portion of the Doppler spectrum as the reference. Note simultaneously displayed plethysmographic tracing (resp) which served for identification of end-expiratory cycles.

The ratio of early to late flow velocity integrals (E/A int) was also assessed. Pressure half time (PHT) of the mitral flow was calculated.[5-9]

Intervals between Q-waves of the ECG and opening and closure of all heart valves were measured either with M-mode echocardiography or pulsed wave Doppler[10] in order to calculate selected systolic and diastolic time intervals of both ventricles. The methodology of measurements and calculations of right heart time intervals was as previously described.[11,12]

Similar methodology was used for measurements of left ventricular time intervals. As duplex M-mode echo provided in many patients the possibility of simultaneous recordings of mitral and aortic valvular events it was considered a method of choice, permitting direct measurements of left ventricular isovolumic relaxation time LVIRT (Fig. 2).

Unfortunately, because of lung hyperinflation, the reliable echo-Doppler assessment of Doppler LV filling indices as well as systolic and diastolic time intervals of both ventricles was possible only in 35 out of 79 studied patients. The patients who remained in the study were divided into those with pulmonary hypertension (PH, n=17) and those with normal pulmonary artery pressure despite chronic lung disease (N, n=18).

Twenty-two out of 35 patients suffered from COPD; in the remaining 13 kyphoscoliosis, pulmonary fibrosis, cystic fibrosis, bronchiectasis or chronic pulmonary thromboembolic disease was diagnosed. Ten age-matched healthy subjects served as controls (HC) providing reference values for echo-Doppler LV

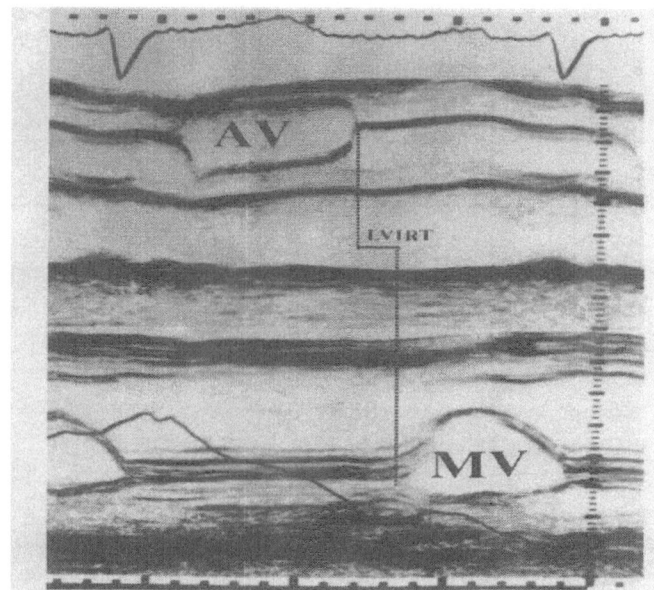

Fig. 2. Simultaneous M-mode tracing of the aortic (AV) and mitral valve (MV) permitting direct measurement of left ventricular relaxation time (LVIRT).

filling indices. The characteristics of the studied population and the parameters analysed are given in tables I and II.

The statistic evaluation consisted of analysis of variance, univariate and multivariate linear regression with stepwise variable selection using the least squares method.

Results

E/A vel ratio was significantly lower in PH than in both N and HC. No difference in E/A vel ratio between N and HC was found (Fig. 3). E/A int was not significantly different between the three groups. PHT was longer in PH than in the two remaining groups (p=0.05), which had PHT of similar duration. LVIRT (corrected for heart rate with Bazett formula i.e. divided by square root of heart cycle length) was slightly longer in PH than in N or HC without reaching statistical significance. None of the Doppler indices of LV filling was statistically different when patients with chronic lung disease irrespective of their pulmonary arterial pressure (PH+N) were compared with healthy controls.

Various parameters showed linear correlations with E/A vel the strongest being those of age, pulmonary arterial pressure (PAP), PaO_2 and right ventricular relaxation time (RVIRT) (Fig. 4). However, no single variable explained more than 42% of the variation of E/A vel. Multivariate stepwise regression analysis using all the available variables was then performed to select best fitting models explaining variations of echo-Doppler LV filling indices (Tabb. III, IV)

The model including RVIRT, DDIAST and Q-AVc was the best fitting one for

Table I. General characteristics of the studied groups

	PH±SD	N±SD	HC±SD
Sex (m/f)	14/3	9/9	7/2
Age (years)	51.7±13.8	46.9±14.1	49.6±14.4
PaO_2 (mmHg)	53.9±15.3 **	73.9±16.6	-
$PaCO_2$ (mmHg)	47.0±8.7 *	40.84±6.6	-
FEV_1 (ml/sec)	1044±699	1280±997	-
HR (bpm)	88.6±16.6	84.8±12.9 **	64.0±9.0
PAP (mmHg)	34.7±11.6 ***	12.9±3.5	-
RAP (mmHg)	3.1±3.3	1.0±3.7	-
Pw (mmHg)	10.1±7.2	5.4±3.7	-

* p<0.05; ** p<0.01; *** p<0.001; SD = standard deviation

Table II. Variables analysed

Haemodynamic (mmHg)

RAP	right atrial mean pressure
RVEDP	right ventricular end-diastolic pressure
PAP	mean pulmonary artery pressure
PASP	pulmonary artery systolic pressure
Pw	pulmonary wedge pressure

Time intervals (msec)

Q-AVc	between Q wave of ECG and	arterial valve closure
Q-PVc	" " " " "	pulmonary valve closure
Q-MVo	" " " " "	mitral valve opening
Q-TVo	" " " " "	tricuspid valve opening
RVIRT	= (Q-TVo) - (Q-PVc)	
LVIRT	= (Q-MVo) - (Q-AVc)	
DDIAST	= LVIRT - RVIRT	
DSYST	= (Q-AVc) - (Q-PVc)	

Echocardiographic (mm)

RVEDD	right ventricular end-diastolic dimension
LVEDD	left ventricular end-diastolic dimension
RV/LV	ratio RVEDD/LVEDD

Other

PaO_2	partial oxygen pressure in the arterialized blood (mmHg)
$PaCO_2$	partial carbon dioxide in the arterialized blood (mmHg)
FEV_1	forced expiratory volumes in 1 sec (ml/sec)
Age	

---

the prediction of E/A vel (R^2 =67%). However, DDIAST showed strong intercorrelation with RVIRT (r=0.82, p<0.001). Moreover, it was composed of RVIRT and LVIRT, the latter being one of the LV diastolic indices. Alternatively RVIRT, age and Q-AVc explained 63% of E/A vel variations (Fig. 5).

According to the regression equation abnormal filling of the left ventricle could be expected if long RVIRT was accompanied by short Q-AVc in an elderly patient. Prolonged PHT coexisted usually with long RVIRT and hypoxaemia, but PHT variations were difficult to predict with available variables (R=40%). E/A integral ratio was abnormal when right ventricular end-diastolic dimension increased with

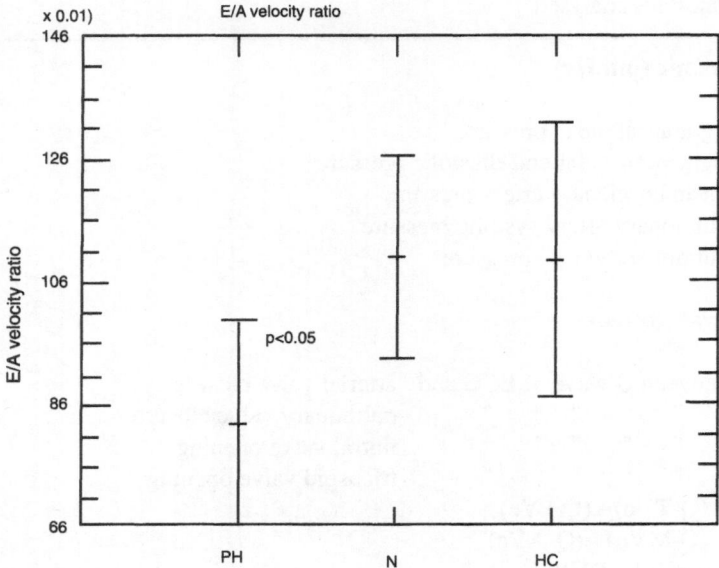

Fig. 3. Mean values and 95% confidence limits for E/A vel ratio in patients with pulmonary hypertension (PH), patients with normal pulmonary artery pressure despite chronic lung disease (N) and in healthy subjects (HC).

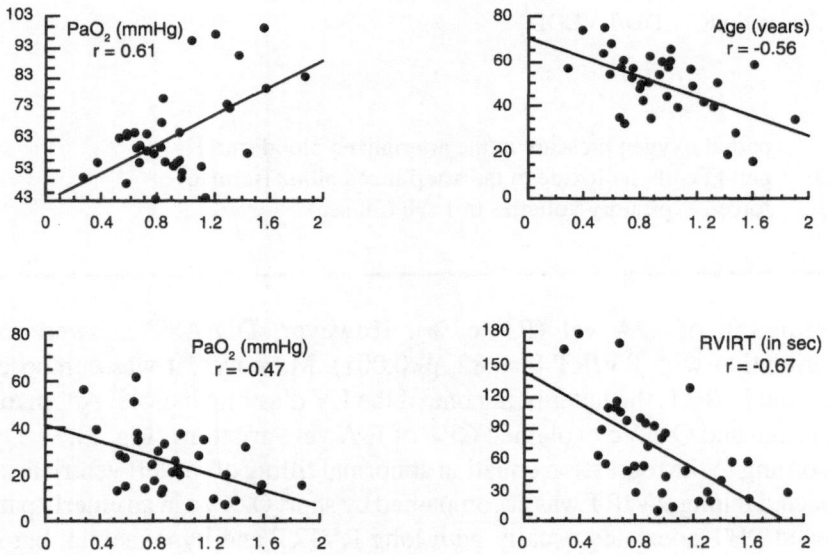

Fig. 4. Correlations between selected variables and E/A vel ratio in 34 patients with chronic lung diseases.

Table III. Echo-Doppler indices of left ventricular filling in patients with (PH) and without pulmonary hypertension (N) and in healthy controls (HC)

	PH±SD		N±SD	HC±SD
E/Avel	0.83±0.33	**	1.10±0.37	1.10±0.23
PHT (msec)	70.8±23.2	*	54.8±16.0	59.1±8.5
E/Aint	1.24±0.76		1.57±0.52	1.66±0.43
LVIRT (msec)	98.9±31.5		84.5±25.1	78.0±25.0

* p=0.05; ** p<0.05 between PH and N

respect to this of the left ventricle in an elderly patient with tachycardia. LVIRT increased either with increasing RVIRT or when right to left ventricular dimension ratio was high in an elderly patient. However, both models resulted in relatively poor LVIRT prediction (R^2 = 30% or 42% respectively).

Discussion

This study analysed four echo-Doppler indices related to the filling pattern of the left ventricle in patients suffering from chronic lung diseases with and without pulmonary hypertension and in normals. Attempts were made to find variables which could be considered responsible for the changes in LV filling patterns

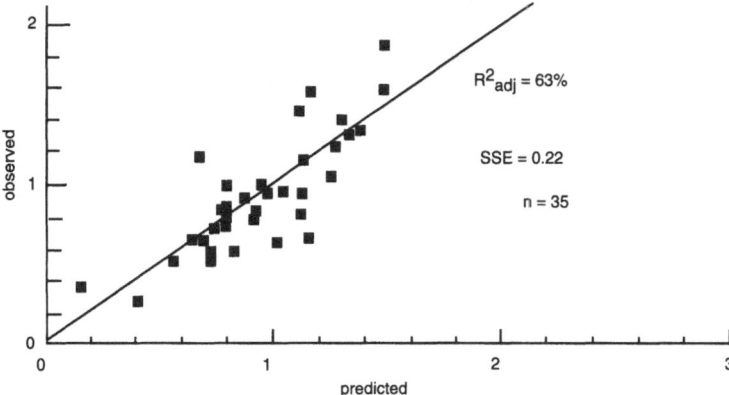

Fig. 5. E/A vel ratio in patients with chronic lung diseases: observed values plotted against values calculated from the multivariate regression equation.

observed in some of the patients. LV diastolic dysfunction was previously described by Louie et al. in patients with primary pulmonary hypertension.[4] They found an inverted relation between early and late diastolic flow and flow velocity as well as prolongation of LVIRT. LV filling impairment was attributed to the leftward displacement of the interventricular septum.

The Authors showed that in the absence of right heart failure or volume overload the septal shift towards the LV cavity was present at end-systole but was most marked in early diastole, with the septum returning toward its normal position and curvature later in diastole. The mechanism of early diastolic leftward shift of the septum was not discussed. Similar early diastolic septal motion abnormalities had been previously observed with M-mode echocardiography in patients with chronic compensated right ventricular pressure overload due to lung disease.[11,13]

However, left ventricular diastolic function was not analysed in these studies. Recently, several communications pointed to abnormal LV diastolic filling in patients with chronic lung diseases. Song et al. found reduced EF slope of mitral echogram in 15 out of 22 patients with cor pulmonale, despite normal coronaries and left ventricular systolic function.[3]

Compared with others, these patients also had an enlarged right ventricle, increased septal thickness and elevated both right and left ventricular end-diastolic pressures. Assayag et al. studied mitral flow velocity pattern in 13 patients with COPD at expiration and inspiration.[2] The E/A vel ratio at inspiration correlated with pulmonary vascular resistance. Pulmonary wedge pressure was elevated but did not correlate with Doppler indices. The Doppler signs of impairment of LV filling during aspiration in patients with COPD were also observed by ourselves (Fig. 6) and by Burghuber (personal communication). On the other hand, similar observations were recently made in healthy children[14] though in normal adults E/A vel ratio

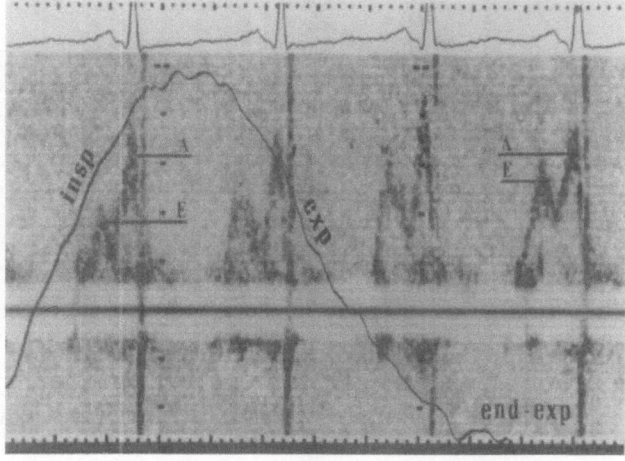

Fig. 6. Effect of respiration on the flow velocity pattern of the mitral valve flow.
E-peak early mitral flow velocity, A-peak mitral flow velocity during atrial contraction.

Table IV. Results of stepwise regression analysis of variables correlating with echo/
Doppler indices of LV filling in 35 patients with chronic lung disease

LV filling index	Variables in the model	R^2adj	SEE	p
E/A vel	RVIRT DDIAST Q-AVc	0.67	0.21	<0.0001
E/A vel	RVIRT Age Q-AVc	0.63	0.22	<0.0001
PHT (msec)	RVIRT PaO$_2$	0.40	16.9	=0.0002
PHT	Age	0.20	19.5	=0.0058
E/A int	Age HR RV/LV	0.52	0.44	<0.0001
LVIRT (msec)	Age RV/LV	0.39	23.2	=0.0002
LVIRT	RVIRT	0.30	24.7	=0.0035

E/A vel = -10^{-4}(71 RVIRT + 49 DDIAST - 48 Q-AVc + 908)
E/A vel = -10^{-4}(33 RVIRT + 58 Age - 38 Q-AVc -2108)
PHT (msec) = 10^{-3}(186 RVIRT + 597 PaO$_2$ + 90191)
PHT (msec) = 0.727 Age + 27.96
E/A int = -10^{-4}(184 Age + 155HR + 7232 RV/LV - 41844)
LVIRT (msec) = 0.76 Age + 40.9 RV/LV
LVIRT (msec) = 0.31 RVIRT + 66.1

was reported to be unaffected by respiration.[15] The causes of changes in left ventricular filling indices during inspiration in patients with chronic lung diseases may be particularly complex due to large variations in the intrathoracic pressure. In the majority of cases systemic venous return increases, leading to higher right heart diastolic pressure and classic ventricular interdependence, but in some patients the opposite may be true because of the collapse of great veins at the entrance to the thorax.[16]

Little is known about pulmonary venous return which might be affected by inspiratory pooling of the blood in the pulmonary vessels and thus decrease left atrial pressure.[16] More importantly, inspiration was shown to increase juxtacardiac pressure, distorting left ventricular geometry and opposing its filling. This external compression of the entire heart may enhance the phenomenon of intraventricular interdependence, with both ventricles competing for the limited space inside the cardiac fossae.[17]

Studying patients with chronic lung disease at relaxed end-expiration during quiet breathing we found abnormal echo-Doppler indices of left ventricular filling only in those subjects who had pulmonary hypertension. Even in this subgroup, only 2 out of 4 studied indices were abnormal (E/A vel, $p<0.05$ and PHT, $p=0.05$). The LV filling pattern was similar in patients with normal pulmonary artery pressure and healthy subjects, despite the difference in heart rates. On the other hand several among the studied variables which included general data, respiratory, haemodynamic and echo-Doppler measurements showed significant correlation with E/Avel ratio found in individual patients (Fig. 5).

None of those variables alone explained more than 42% of variation of E/A vel. Intercorrelation between some of those variables made it difficult to assess their relative significance in the pathophysiology of LV diastolic filling.

Stepwise multivariate regression analysis disclosed that various indices of LV filling correlated with different sets of variables. The variables which entered regression equations predicting four different echo-Doppler indices of LV filling could be divided into three categories: RVIRT, PaO_2 and RV/LV could be regarded as consequences of chronic lung disease.

Age was independent and Q-AVc and heart rate were non-specific parameters, though possibly affected by chronic lung disease. Of all studied variables age and RVIRT were most often represented in regression equations and had highest partial statistical significance. The influence of age on left ventricular diastolic function is well recognized.[18,19,20]

RVIRT seems to be the most important determinant of LV filling which might be related to chronic lung disease. It is tempting to speculate that prolonged relaxation of the right ventricle might result in momentary inversion of the pressures on both sides of the interventricular septum, explaining abnormal septal position impeding early left ventricular filling as observed by Louie et al.

Unfortunately, we were not able to obtain good quality short axis images of the left ventricle in many of our patients, and the relation of prolonged RVIRT and abnormal septal position in early diastole could not be directly confirmed. RVIRT prolongation is probably due to several factors, some of which result from chronic lung disease.

Apart from increased pulmonary arterial pressure which is a well recognized cause of RVIRT prolongation[11,12,21,22] it seems likely that it might be affected by right ventricular hypertrophy, ischaemia (or hypoxaemia) or myocardial fibrosis.[23] In fact we found correlations between RVIRT and PAP ($r = 0.60$), PaO_2 ($r = 0.44$) and age ($r=0.42$).

The lack of catheterization laboratory data among the variables selected for multivariate regressions is interesting. It should be remembered, that right heart catheterization was performed within 1-2 days of the non-invasive echo-Doppler studies, the latter being practically simultaneous with evaluation of LV filling indices. Stress should finally be put on the fact that the study could not provide direct evidence of the causative relationship between measured variables and LV filling indices. Moreover, echo-Doppler, though recognized as a convenient method for non-invasive assessment of the diastolic ventricular function, has its own limitations, discussion of which exceeds the scope of this paper.[6,9]

In conclusion we found abnormalities in two (E/Avel, PHT) out of four echo Doppler indices of LV filling in those patients with chronic lung disease who had pulmonary hypertension. Multivariate analysis identified variables which might be responsible for LV filling pattern in patients suffering from chronic lung disease, with right ventricular relaxation time and age apparently being the most important ones. Prolongation of RVIRT is mainly a result of pulmonary hypertension but a contribution may be expected also from other factors such as right ventricular hypertrophy, myocardial ischaemia/hypoxaemia or fibrosis.

It is suggested that prolonged RVIRT might invert early diastolic pressures on both sides of the interventricular septum, leading to septal displacement, left ventricular distortion and early diastolic filling impairment which we observed during relaxed expiration in patients with pulmonary hypertension due to chronic diseases.

References

1. Morpurgo M., Denolin H.: The heart in pulmonary hypertension due to lung disease. In: Wagenvoort C.A., Denolin H. (Eds.) *Pulmonary Circulation*. Amsterdam, Elsevier Science Publishers BV 1989; p. 163-189
2. Assayag P., Brochet E., Faraggi M., Mal H., Gamerman G., Pariente R., Valere P.E.: Left ventricular filling impairment in chronic obstructive lung disease with right ventricular pressure overload. (abstr). Eur. Heart J. 1989; 10-8
3. Song G.J., Jones C.J.H., Oldershaw P.J.: Mechanism of left ventricular diastolic dysfunction in cor pulmonale - the role of interventricular transmission of raised right ventricular pressure (abstr). Eur. Heart J. 1989; 10-8
4. Louie E.K., Rich S., Brundage B.H.: Doppler echocardiographic assessment of impaired left ventricular filling in patients with right ventricular pressure overload due to pulmonary hypertension. Am. J. Cardiol. 1986; 8:1298-1306
5. Rokey R., Kuo L.C., Zoghbi W.A., Limacher M.C., Quinones M.A.: Determination of parameters of diastolic filling with pulsed Doppler echocardiography: comparison with cineangiography. Circulation 1985; 71:543-550
6. Snider A.R., Gidding S.S., Rocchini A.P., Rosenthal A., Dick M., Crowley D.C., Peters J.: Doppler evaluation of left ventricular diastolic filling in children with systemic hypertension. Am. J. Cardiol. 1985; 56:921-926
7. Hatle L.K., Angelsen B.: *Doppler ultrasound in cardiology: physical principles and clinical*

applications. Philadelphia, Lea and Febiger, 2nd edition, 1985
8. Labovitz A.J., Williams G.A.: *Doppler Echocardiography. The Quantitative Approach.* Philadelphia, Lea and Febiger 1989; p. 85-100
9. Appleton C.P., Hatle L.K., Popp R.L.: Relation of transmitral flow velocity patterns to left ventricular diastolic function. New insights from a combined hemodynamic and Doppler echocardiographic study. J. Am. Coll. Cardiol. 1988; 12:426-440
10. Hsieh K.S., Sanders S.P., Colan S.D., MacPherson D., Holland C.: Right ventricular systolic time intervals: comparison of echocardiographic and Doppler derived values. Am. Heart J. 1986; 112:103-106
11. Torbicki A., Hawrylkiewicz I., Zielinski J.: Value of M-mode echocardiography in assessing pulmonary arterial pressure in patients with chronic lung disease. Bull. Eur. Physiopathol. Respir. 1987; 23:233-239
12. Torbicki A., Skwarski K., Hawrylkiewicz I., Pasierski T., Miskiewicz Z., Zielinski J.: Attempts at measuring pulmonary arterial pressure with Doppler echocardiography in patients with chronic lung diseases. Eur. Respir. J. 1989
13. Morpurgo M., Saviotti M., Dickele M.C., Casazza F., Torbicki A., Weitzenblum E., Zielinski J.: Echocardiographic aspects of pulmonary hypertension in chronic lung disease. Bull. Eur. Physiopath. Respir. 1984; 20: 251-255
14. Riggs T.W., Snider A.R.: Respiratory influence on RV and LV diastolic filling in normal children (abstr). J. Am. Coll. Cardiol. 1989; 13: 205A
15. Uiterval C., Van Dam I., De Boo Th., Van Keulen P., Folgering H., Hopman J., Daniels O.: The effect of respiration on diastolic blood flow velocities in the human heart. Eur. Heart. J. 1989; 10:108-112
16. Scharf S.M.: Effects of normal and stressed inspiration on cardiovascular function. In: Scharf S.M., Cassidy S.S. (Eds) *Heart-lung interactions in health and disease* New York, Basel, Marcel Dekker Inc. 1989; p. 427-461
17. Lloyd T.C.: Mechanical heart-lung interactions. In: Scharf S.M., Cassidy S.S. (Eds) *Heart-lung interactions in health and disease.* New York-Basel, Marcel Dekker, 1989; p. 309-336
18. Miyatake K., Okamoto M., Kinoshita N., Owa M., Nakasone I., Sakakibara H., Nimura Y.: Augmentation of atrial contribution to left ventricular inflow with ageing as assessed by intracardiac Doppler flowmetry. Am. J. Cardiol. 1984; 53:586-589
19. Miller T.R., Grossman S.J., Schectman K.B., Biello D.R., Ludbrook P.A., Ehsani A.A.: Left ventricular diastolic filling and its association with age. Am. J. Cardiol. 1986; 58:531-535
20. Kuo L.C., Quinones M.A., Rokey R., Sartori M., Abinader E.G., Zoghbi W.A.: Quantification of atrial contribution to left ventricular filling by pulsed Doppler echocardiography and the effect of age in normal and diseased hearts. Am. J. Cardiol. 1987; 59:1174-1178
21. Burstin L.: Determination of pressure in the pulmonary artery by external graphic recordings. Br. Heart J. 1967; 29:396-404
22. Hatle L., Angelsen B.A.J., Tromsdal A.: Noninvasive estimation of pulmonary artery systolic pressure with Doppler ultrasound. Br. Heart J. 1981; 45:157-165
23. Triffon D., Groves B.M., Reeves J.T., Ditchey R.V.: Determinants of the relation between systolic pressure and duration of isovolumic relaxation in the right ventricle. J. Am. Coll. Cardiol. 1988; 11:322-329

Subject Index

I

L

M